Complications in Orthopaedics
Anterior Cruciate Ligament Surgery

Edited by
Kevin B. Freedman, MD, MSCE
Attending Orthopaedic Surgeon
Orthopaedic Specialists
Bryn Mawr, Pennsylvania

Series Editor
Jeffrey O. Anglen, MD
Professor and Chairman
Department of Orthopaedics
Indiana University School of Medicine
Indianapolis, Indiana

Published by the
American Academy of Orthopaedic Surgeons
6300 North River Road
Rosemont, IL 60018

American Academy of Orthopaedic Surgeons

Staff
Mark Wieting, *Chief Education Officer*
Marilyn L. Fox, PhD, *Director, Department of Publications*
Lynne Roby Shindoll, *Managing Editor*
Joan Abern, *Senior Editor*
Mary Steermann, *Manager, Production and Archives*
Sophie Tosta, *Assistant Production Manager*
Susan Morritz Baim, *Production Coordinator*
Karen Danca, *Production Assistant*
Anne Raci, *Page Production Assistant*

American Academy of Orthopaedic Surgeons
6300 North River Road
Rosemont, IL 60018
1-800-626-6726

First Edition

ISBN 0-89203-366-5

Bone and Joint DECADE 2002 - USA - 2011

Contributors

Bernard R. Bach, Jr, MD
The Claude N. Lambert-Helen S. Thompson Professor of Orthopaedic Surgery
Director, Division of Sports Medicine
Department of Orthopaedic Surgery
Rush Medical College of Rush University
Chicago, Illinois

Charles A. Bush-Joseph, MD
Associate Professor
Department of Orthopaedic Surgery
Rush Medical College of Rush University
Chicago, Illinois

Mitchell Fagelman, MD
Department of Orthopaedic Surgery
Loyola University Medical Center
Stritch School of Medicine
Maywood, Illinois

Kyle R. Flik, MD
Sports Medicine
Northeast Orthopaedics, LLP
Albany, New York

Kevin B. Freedman, MD, MSCE
Attending Orthopaedic Surgeon
Orthopaedic Specialists
Bryn Mawr, Pennsylvania

Michael Garcia, MD
Division of Sports Medicine
Department of Orthopaedic Surgery
Stritch School of Medicine
Loyola University Health Systems
Maywood, Illinois

Ronald Edward Glenn, Jr, MD
Fellow
Division of Sports Medicine
Department of Orthopaedic Surgery
Rush Medical College of Rush University
Chicago, Illinois

Jeffrey J. Kovacic, MD
Orthopaedic Sports Fellow
Cleveland Clinic Sports Health
Department of Orthopaedic Surgery
The Cleveland Clinic Foundation
Cleveland, Ohio

Richard D. Parker, MD
Education Director
Cleveland Clinic Sports Health
Department of Orthopaedic Surgery
The Cleveland Clinic Foundation
Cleveland, Ohio

Contributors

Randall J. Risinger, MD
Fellow
Division of Sports Medicine
Department of Orthopaedic Surgery
Rush Medical College of Rush
University
Chicago, Illinois

Harold Schock, MD
Department of Orthopaedic Surgery
Stritch School of Medicine
Loyola University Health Systems
Maywood, Illinois

Kurt P. Spindler, MD
Vice-Chairman and Professor
Department of Orthopaedics
Vanderbilt University Medical Center
Nashville, Tennessee

Pietro Tonino, MD
Division of Sports Medicine
Department of Orthopaedic Surgery
Stritch School of Medicine
Loyola University Health Systems
Maywood, Illinois

Contents

Preface vii

1 Intraoperative Complications: Graft Harvest 1

2 Intraoperative Complications: Graft Fixation Problems 9

3 Extensor Mechanism Compromise and Patellar Fracture 21

4 Septic Arthritis Following ACL Reconstruction 29

5 Arthrofibrosis Following ACL Reconstruction 35

6 Failed ACL Reconstruction: Evaluation for Revision ACL Reconstruction 49

7 Technical Aspects for Revision ACL Reconstruction 61

Index 75

Preface

An estimated 80,000 anterior cruciate ligament (ACL) injuries occur annually in the United States. For most young, athletic patients, ACL reconstruction is recommended to stabilize the knee and protect the meniscus and articular cartilage from further damage. ACL reconstruction has been shown to restore stability to the knee in more than 90% of patients. However, given the large number of ACL reconstructions performed annually, complications inevitably are encountered.

Despite the abundance of literature on both the basic science and surgical outcomes of ACL reconstruction, little has been written about the management of complications from ACL reconstruction. A complication can be defined as an unexpected event that occurs during the course of treatment, whereas a failure is an unsuccessful result of treatment. The goal of this monograph is to help the reader prevent common complications related to ACL reconstruction but also to quickly identify and manage them when they occur. Our goal should be to prevent every complication from becoming a treatment failure.

Although ACL reconstruction is a commonly performed operation with highly successful results, a high level of technical detail is required to optimize the results. The first two chapters of this monograph focus on how to identify and manage intraoperative complications when they arise.

Bone-patellar tendon-bone and quadrupled hamstrings autografts are the most commonly used grafts for ACL reconstruction. Both restore knee stability and function with strength that surpasses that of the native ACL. However, a successful graft harvest is essential to optimizing the postoperative outcome. Each type of graft has unique complications that can occur during harvest. Charles Bush-Joseph, MD, and his colleagues emphasize the importance of preoperative planning to address potential complications and to ensure adequate graft material for reconstruction.

Complications in graft fixation also can occur; therefore, alternative fixation methods must be planned. The most common problem associated with femoral fixation is posterior wall blowout. Harold Schock, MD, and I describe this complication and other graft fixation problems for both patellar tendon and hamstrings autografts in chapter 2.

Several complications associated with ACL reconstruction can be devastating; therefore, a chapter is dedicated to each major complication. I asked Bernard Bach, MD, and several of his colleagues to address postoperative extensor mechanism compromise or injury in chapter 3 and, although rare, arthrofibrosis in chapter 5. The former is more common with patellar tendon autografts, but anterior knee pain following ACL reconstruction can occur with all graft types. The latter can be severely debilitating if not aggressively managed in the early postoperative period. In chapter 4, Kurt Spindler, MD, and associates supply an excellent discussion of septic arthritis, also a rare but debilitating complication of ACL reconstruction.

Finally, despite all attempts to ensure a successful outcome, ACL failure does occur. The final two chapters of the monograph describe the evaluation and management of the failed ACL reconstruction, including revision ACL reconstruction. Mitchell Fagelman, MD, and I describe the evaluation for revision ACL reconstruction, and Dr. Bach and Ron Glenn, MD, provide an excellent and highly detailed discussion of the technical aspects of revision ACL surgery.

This monograph series on complications is unique in that each chapter is presented in a case-based format. Each chapter begins with the history and initial management of the patient. The next section describes the complication, including recognition of the problem, management options, and strategies for preventing the problem. The chapter closes with a report of the final case management and outcome summary.

All orthopaedic surgeons treating patients with ACL injuries, including residents and fellows in training, practicing general orthopaedic surgeons, and experienced sports medicine specialists, should find this monograph informative. It provides a comprehensive treatment approach to many of the complications that will occur following ACL reconstruction.

I was fortunate to assemble a group of highly respected and experienced national experts on ACL reconstruction and sincerely thank them for their contributions. Their insights on the management of each problem lay the foundation for this monograph. I especially wish to thank them for their contributions of artwork, particularly the excellent case studies and clear illustrations of technique. These have added much to this discussion. I would like to thank Jeffrey Anglen, MD, for his oversight and excellent suggestions on the manuscript. I also would like to thank the AAOS Publications Department, especially Joan Abern, Senior Editor, Lynne Shindoll, Managing Editor, and Sophie Tosta, Assistant Production Manager, for all of their efforts in bringing this project to publication.

Kevin B. Freedman, MD, MSCE
Editor

Chapter 1

Intraoperative Complications: Graft Harvest

Kyle R. Flik, MD
Charles A. Bush-Joseph, MD

Case Presentations

Case 1

Patella Tendon Harvest: Inadequate Bone Plug

History

A 20-year-old male college soccer player presented with an unstable right knee after a noncontact injury that occurred during a game. Physical examination 5 days after his injury revealed a slightly antalgic gait and moderate knee effusion. He had a 10° loss of extension and a 15° loss of flexion compared to his contralateral knee. He also had a grade IIB Lachman test and a positive pivot-shift test. MRI revealed a midsubstance tear of the anterior cruciate ligament (ACL) and a lateral meniscus tear (**Figure 1**).

Physical therapy was prescribed three times a week for 4 weeks to restore range of motion and strength. After this 4-week period, full range of motion was restored and there was no swelling, although the patient reported persistent instability. At this follow-up appointment, graft choices were discussed, including the advantages and disadvantages of bone-patellar tendon-bone (BTB) autograft, hamstring autograft, and allograft. The patient and surgeon elected to use the BTB autograft. Traditionally, this graft choice is recommended for competitive athletes involved in level 1 sports that require cutting and sharp pivoting maneuvers.

Current Problem and Treatment

The graft harvest was initiated using an incision just medial to the midline, which allowed access to both the tibial tubercle and the superior pole of the patella. The paratenon was then incised and preserved. A 10-mm patellar tendon graft was cut from the central third of the tendon. The tibial bone plug (10 × 25 mm) was harvested using an oscillating saw. During its extrication with an osteotome, the bone plug fractured, leaving only a minimal amount of bone attached to the tendon. The remainder of the harvest proceeded as planned with

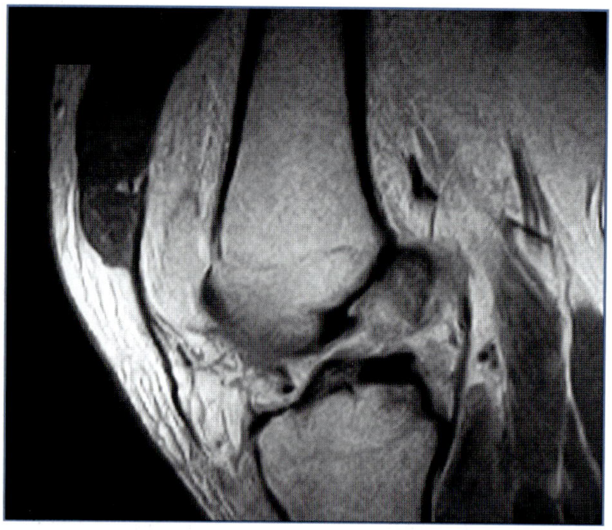

Figure 1 Sagittal MRI scan showing a midsubstance tear of the ACL.

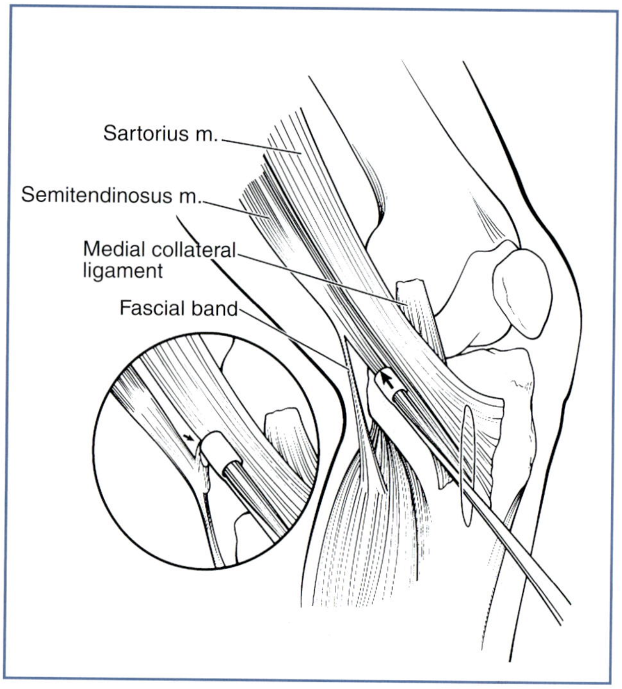

Figure 2 Medial side of the knee with inset shows the tendon stripper advancing and prematurely cutting the semitendinosus tendon, which is tethered by a fascial band at the arrow.

uneventful removal of the bone plug from the patella. However, the patellar tendon harvest resulted in a bone block that was inadequate for fixation.

Case 2

Hamstring Tendon Harvest: Premature Graft Amputation

History

A 19-year-old female ballet dancer with a history of chronic anterior knee pain and patellar tendinitis presented with an acute painful hemarthrosis after landing awkwardly from a jump. The patient, who is 5'6" and weighs 110 lb, was diagnosed with a ruptured ACL based on a positive pivot-shift test and grade IIB Lachman test on physical examination. MRI confirmed the diagnosis.

ACL reconstruction with a hamstrings autograft was scheduled after 6 weeks of physical therapy to restore motion and strength in the knee. A hamstrings autograft was selected because the patient's small patella and patellar tendon may have resulted in a narrow central-third graft and because of the risk of extensor mechanism morbidity associated with obtaining this type of graft, especially given her history of patellar tendinitis.

Current Problem and Treatment

Examination under anesthesia was unequivocal; therefore, hamstrings tendon harvest was initiated before arthroscopy. A 3-cm incision was made medial to the tibial tubercle, and then the pes anserinus and sartorial fascial expansion were incised. The gracilis tendon was removed without difficulty using an open-ended tendon stripper; however, during removal of the semitendinosus tendon, the graft was unexpectedly truncated, yielding only 10 cm of tendon. A large fibrous band tethering the semitendinosus tendon was unrecognized, which caused the tendon stripper to divert its course while being advanced by the surgeon; thus, the tendon was prematurely cut (**Figure 2**). The result was the potential for insufficient graft material for ACL reconstruction.

Discussion

Patellar Tendon Harvest

Intraoperative complications during the harvest of a BTB graft may include inadequate tendon or bone plug size, patellar fracture, and various forms of donor site morbidity, including extensor mechanism disruption.[1]

The BTB graft should be obtained, as described by Bach and associates,[2] using careful surgical technique with adequate exposure. The full width of the patellar tendon should be measured before harvest to ensure that both the harvested portion and the remaining tendon are adequate because a narrow patellar tendon (< 30 mm) may require the use of a smaller central-third graft (< 10 mm) or a substitute graft. The knee should be placed in flexion when cutting the tendon to put tension on the fibers and promote a straight longitudinal cut. Cutting with the knee in extension allows laxity in the tendon and may lead to an inadvertent cut across the longitudinal fibers, resulting in graft compromise or disruption of the remaining patellar tendon. Care is needed to clearly define and remove only the central third of the patellar tendon to avoid postoperative rupture of the remaining two thirds.

A small or fragmented bone plug may result from attempting to remove the plug before adequately completing the bone cuts with the oscillating saw, especially in the corners of the cut (**Figure 3**, *A*). Should this complication occur, a tendon-securing Krackow stitch with nonabsorbable suture can be placed around the tendon and into any remaining bone[1] (**Figure 3**, *B*). This portion of the graft can be secured either using soft-tissue interference fixation (metal or bioabsorbable soft-tissue interference screw) or simply tying it around a screw and post on the tibia. If sufficient bone remains on the graft, the bone plug can be augmented by piggybacking bone obtained from a coring reamer onto the bone plug and attaching the two with suture through drill holes (**Figure 3**, *C* and *D*).

If the bone plug is grossly undersized, interference fixation may not be possible. For femur-sided fixation, soft-tissue fixation methods, such as the EndoButton CL (Smith & Nephew Endoscopy, Andover, MA) or cross-pin fixation can be used. Another option is to undersize the femoral tunnel to match the small bone plug and then proceed with interference fixation.

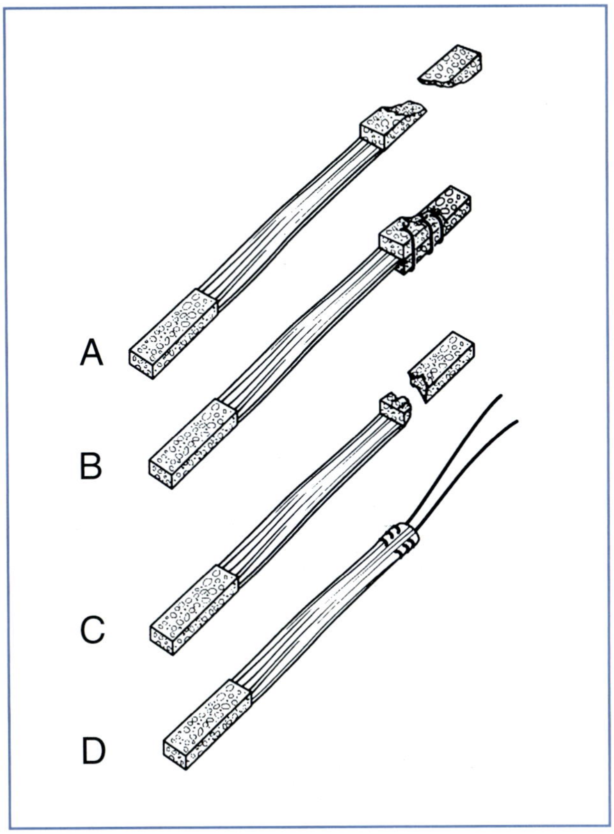

Figure 3 **A**, Fractured bone plug with a significant amount of bone intact. **B**, Proposed solution to a fractured bone plug using a bone graft piggyback technique. **C**, BTB autograft with damaged and inadequate bone plug. **D**, Removal of all remaining bone and conversion to a soft-tissue graft technique.

An oscillating saw should be used to obtain a patellar plug that is from 20- to 25-mm long, 9- to 10-mm wide, and approximately 6- to 7-mm deep, with beveled cuts along the patellar surface.[2] Knowing the total length of the oscillating saw blade is helpful to gauge its depth during the cuts. If complete cuts are made, then minimal use of an osteotome should be required to gently remove the plug. An additional measure to preserve extensor mechanism strength involves angling the block cut in the tibia to leave a triangular trough, which maximizes the bone stock beneath the remaining patellar tendon attachments (**Figure 4**).

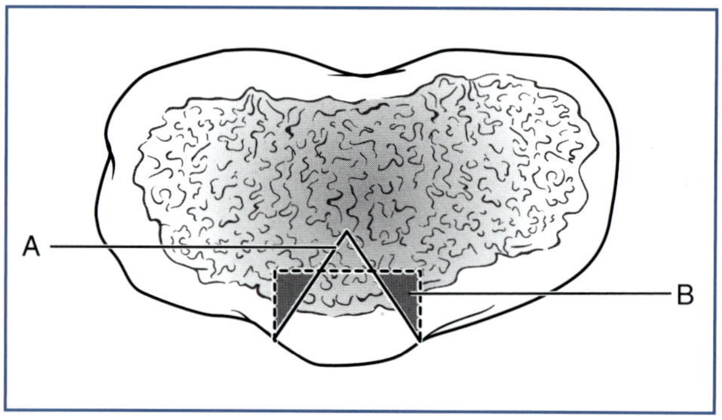

Figure 4 Cross-section of the proximal tibia at the level of patellar tendon insertion. Note that angling the cut as shown (A) preserves bone (shaded area), leaving a rectangular area of bone stock (B) at the central-third patellar insertion.

Most patellar fractures in the ACL-reconstructed knee occur postoperatively; however, intraoperative fractures do occur.[3] The management of these fractures is discussed in a separate chapter.

Other potential pitfalls during harvest of a BTB graft are associated with morbidity at the donor site, most of which is preventable, specifically: (1) cooling the oscillating blade with water may minimize thermal necrosis of bone or skin; (2) using the osteotome carefully and gently can avoid chondral damage to the articular surface of the patella or trochlea; and (3) repairing the preserved vascular paratenon during closure can maximize the healing potential of the remaining patellar tendon. Although we recommend bone grafting of the patellar defect using a technique described by Ferrari and Bach,[4] doing so has not been proved to significantly affect clinical or functional outcomes.[5]

Hamstrings Tendon Harvest

Mastering the anatomy on the medial side of the knee will help prevent most of the more common pitfalls that may occur during harvest of the semitendinosus and gracilis tendons (**Figure** 5). These tendons are located between layer 1 (sartorius fascia) and layer 2 (superficial medial collateral ligament [MCL]) on the medial side of the knee.[6] The sartorius tendon is superficial to the gracilis and semitendinosus tendons and proximal to their insertion, but it fuses with these tendons distally to form the pes anserinus, which inserts onto the proximal anteromedial tibia.

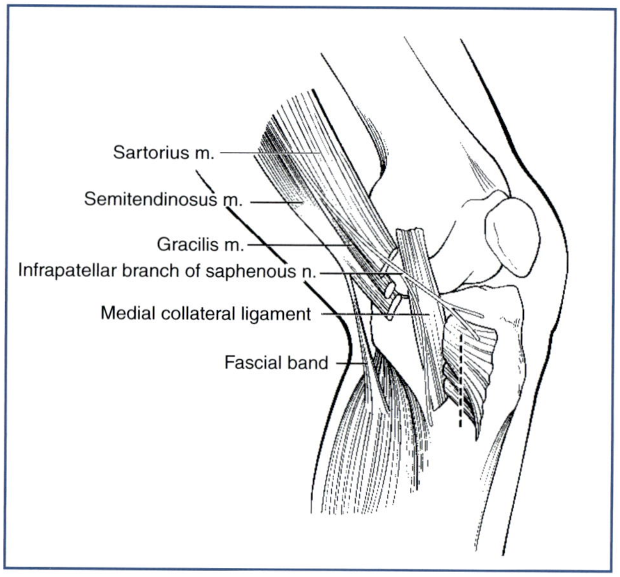

Figure 5 Relevant anatomy on the medial side of the knee. Note that during harvest of the hamstrings tendon, use of a longitudinal incision (dotted line) provides better exposure for drilling the tibial tunnel.

Solman and Pagnani[7] described the anatomic relationships in this region. The pes anserinus insertion is an average of 19 mm distal and 22.5 mm medial to the apex of the tibial tubercle and has an average width of 20 mm. At a point 18 mm proximal to the common insertion, the gracilis (superior and more round) and semitendinosus (inferior and flatter) become separate and distinct structures beneath the sartorius fascia. The superficial MCL is deep to the tendons in this area.

The first potential complication that can be encountered during hamstrings tendon harvest is injury to the infrapatellar branch of the saphenous nerve as a result of the incision.[8] An oblique or transverse incision is more likely to avoid this common pitfall; however, we prefer a longitudinal incision with cautious dissection through the subcutaneous tissues because it provides better exposure for drilling the tibial tunnel (Figure 5).

After the gracilis and semitendinosus tendons are located, they should be isolated proximally toward their musculotendinous junction, and all adhesions

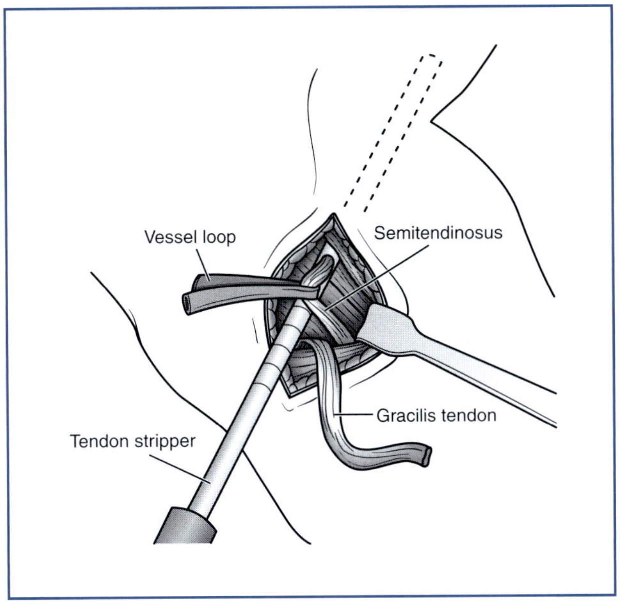

Figure 6 Use of the tendon stripper.

and accessory bands dissected. These fascial bands, usually 8 to 10 cm proximal to the pes anserinus, are dense and adhere to the gracilis and semitendinosus tendons, which could potentially cause inadvertent truncation of the graft during stripping, as shown in Figure 2. The semitendinosus may have up to five accessory bands or insertions that must be released for the tendon stripper to pass unencumbered over the tendon. The tendon stripper is advanced with the patient's leg in the figure-of-four position and the stripper aimed along the direction of the muscle's origin (**Figure 6**). This leg position gives direct access for the tendon stripper to be advanced and also decreases tension on the saphenous nerve, minimizing the risk of damage.

A dreaded pitfall of hamstrings tendon stripping is premature graft amputation,[7] but it can be avoided with complete understanding of hamstrings anatomy and proper use of the tendon stripper. Complete, careful dissection of all fascial bands and accessory insertions from the gracilis and semitendinosus tendons is emphasized. If, despite folding the tendons over on themselves to create a collagen bundle, sufficient tissue is not obtained to create an adequately stout graft, an alternative graft source should be considered (ie, quadriceps tendon[9] or allograft[10]). An undersized graft is not acceptable. A 7- to 8-mm graft generally is the smallest diameter that we would accept in a patient with a small knee and slight build, such as the patient in the second case study. At times, a graft of this size can be achieved by suturing three graft limbs together side by side. If the tendon is truncated far distally, it may be feasible to explore for the cut tendon edge and complete the stripping process proximally to obtain the remainder of the tendon. However, in our experience attempted salvage of a truncated hamstrings graft usually is not successful, and an alternate graft choice is made.

Exposure of the gracilis and semitendinosus places the underlying tendons or the superficial MCL at risk, either of which can be damaged if the surgeon plunges with the scalpel when incising the sartorius fascia. It is important to avoid mistaking the MCL for one of the hamstring tendons. Other uncommon but reported complications from hamstrings harvest include sciatic nerve damage[11] and thigh hematoma (SJ O'Brien, MD, personal communication, 2003).

Graft Contamination

The possibility of graft contamination is ubiquitous, regardless of the type of graft used and despite the use of standard sterile procedures. Contamination usually is the result of human error, such as dropping the graft because of carelessness during transport. To avoid this catastrophe, the graft should not be passed from person to person. The surgeon should always transport the graft after harvesting is complete, communicate with all members of the surgical team regarding the location of the graft, and retrieve the graft when it is needed.

We recommend obtaining an alternate graft source whenever possible if loss of sterility occurs for any reason. Sterilization techniques using 4% chlorhexidine followed by a triple-antibiotic solution are reported to provide 100% sterility in a controlled in vivo rabbit model;[12] therefore, this sterilization method is preferred if an alternative graft source is not available. This method requires soaking the graft in 4% chlorhexidine gluconate for 30 minutes, followed by a soaking in triple-antibiotic solution for another 30 minutes, and then a brief rinse in saline solution. Although contamination of a procured autograft is unusual, alternative graft sources should be available in all ACL reconstructions in anticipation of potential contamination.

Ideally, a surgeon performing an ACL reconstruction should be comfortable and adept at harvesting BTB and hamstrings grafts or using allograft tissue, if needed. Preoperatively, the surgeon should discuss with patients the possibility of requiring alternate grafts during ACL reconstruction.

Management and Outcome Summary

Case 1

Patellar Tendon Harvest: Inadequate Bone Plug

The solution for the first patient was to completely remove the remaining bone and use soft-tissue fixation on the tibial side of the graft. In this way, we essentially converted a BTB graft into a graft similar to an Achilles allograft with a single bone plug for the femoral side. We did not use the piggyback technique of adding a bone graft to the small bone plug, which is a better solution when there is a solid but undersized bone plug to which additional bone can be secured easily. In this case, we believed that the remaining bone was inadequate for standard interference fixation, which is an additional option when the bone plug is compromised but retains sufficient size and quality to support an interference screw.

The patient tolerated the procedure well and had an uneventful postoperative course. He worked diligently at rehabilitation and returned to competitive soccer 8 months postoperatively.

Case 2

Hamstrings Tendon Harvest: Premature Amputation

In the second case, in which premature cutting of the semitendinosus occurred during hamstrings harvest, the management options were more limited. We could use the available tendons, augment them, or choose an alternative graft. The total amount of collagen was immediately assessed to determine if a sufficient graft could be formed from the available hamstrings tendons. Although we routinely fashion hamstrings grafts into a quadrupled structure, this particular graft was not long enough; therefore, we created a tripled construct.

We considered the patient's slight build and small bone structure when assessing the adequacy of the harvest. The patient was a petite woman with a small knee for whom we believed a 7-mm graft would suffice; we would not have accepted a smaller graft. Once prepared, the tripled hamstrings graft fit well into a 7-mm cylindrical tube. The graft was then fixed on the femoral side of the knee with a bioabsorbable interference screw; it was fixed on the tibial side with a bioabsorbable interference screw and supplemented with suture over a post for back-up fixation.

The patient did well and was last seen at her 3-month follow-up visit where she had no complaints and was proceeding with physical therapy without difficulties. She had a normal Lachman test and no pivot shift.

The only remaining options would have been to harvest the contralateral hamstrings to augment the graft, to use ipsilateral or contralateral BTB, or to use an allograft. All of these options require proper informed consent.

Strategies to Minimize Common Complications

For patellar tendon harvest, it is important when removing bone plugs in either the tibia or the patella to fully complete the corner cuts with the oscillating saw before attempting to remove the plug with an osteotome. Angling the blade 45° when making the transverse cut helps to achieve this.

We previously described the proper way to prevent prematurely cutting the hamstrings tendons during harvest. To summarize, it is crucial to adequately visualize the tendons as far proximally as possible and to release all accessory fibrous bands or adhesions before using the tendon stripper. The tendon stripper should point toward the tendon origin while the surgeon is pushing proximally with steady pressure.

In addition, alternate graft choices always should be discussed with the patient preoperatively when obtaining informed consent. This step will help accommodate a graft choice change caused by intraoperative problems.

References

1. Cain EL Jr, Gillogly SD, Andrews JR:Management of intraoperative complications associated with autogenous patellar tendon graft anterior cruciate ligament reconstruction. *Instr Course Lect* 2003;52:359-367.
2. Bach BR Jr, Levy ME, Bojchuk J, Tradonsky S, Bush-Joseph CA, Khan NH: Single-incision endoscopic anterior cruciate ligament reconstruction using patellar tendon autograft: Minimum two-year follow-up evaluation. *Am J Sports Med* 1998;26:30-40.
3. Berg EE: Management of patella fractures associated with central third bone-patella tendon-bone autograft ACL reconstructions. *Arthroscopy* 1996;12:756-759.
4. Ferrari JD, Bach BR Jr: Bone graft procurement for patellar defect grafting in anterior cruciate ligament reconstruction. *Arthroscopy* 1998;14:543-545.
5. Brandsson S, Faxen E, Eriksson BI, et al: Closing patellar tendon defects after anterior cruciate ligament reconstruction: Absence of any benefit. *Knee Surg Sports Traumatol Arthrosc* 1998;6:82-87.
6. Warren LF, Marshall JL: The supporting structures and layers on the medial side of the knee: An anatomical analysis. *J Bone Joint Surg Am* 1979;61:56-62.
7. Solman CG Jr, Pagnani MJ: Hamstring tendon harvesting: Reviewing anatomic relationships and avoiding pitfalls. *Orthop Clin North Am* 2003;34:1-8.
8. Mochizuki T, Akita K, Minneta T, Sato T: Anatomic bases for minimizing sensory disturbance after arthroscopically-assisted anterior cruciate ligament reconstruction using medial hamstring tendons. *Surg Radiol Anat* 2003;25:192-199.
9. Antonogiannakis E, Yiannakopoulos CK, Hiotis I, Karabalis C, Babalis G: Arthroscopic anterior cruciate ligament reconstruction using quadriceps tendon autograft and bioabsorbable cross-pin fixation. *Arthroscopy* 2005;21:894.
10. Kustos T, Balint L, Than P, Bardos T: Comparative study of autograft or allograft in primary anterior cruciate ligament reconstruction. *Int Orthop* 2004;28:290-293.
11. Vardi G: Sciatic nerve injury following hamstring harvest. *Knee* 2004;11:37-39.
12. Goebel ME, Drez D Jr, Heck SB, Stoma MK: Contaminated rabbit patellar tendon grafts: In vivo analysis of disinfecting methods. *Am J Sports Med* 1994;22:387-391.

Chapter 2

Intraoperative Complications: Graft Fixation Problems

Harold Schock, MD
Kevin B. Freedman, MD, MSCE

Case Presentation

History

A 19-year-old female collegiate basketball player sustained a twisting injury to her right knee when she landed from a rebound. She reported that she heard a pop as she landed and described immediate development of an effusion. Physical examination in the office 2 weeks later revealed a grade IIB Lachman test, no joint line tenderness, and full active and passive range of motion. MRI showed an acute anterior cruciate ligament (ACL) tear with pivot-shift contusions but no meniscal tears (**Figure 1**). She was highly motivated to return to sports as soon as possible.

Current Problem and Treatment

Three weeks after the injury, the patient underwent a central-third bone-patellar tendon-bone (BTB) autograft ACL reconstruction. During the procedure, a 7-mm femoral offset guide was placed in the over-the-top position in preparation for femoral drilling. A Beath pin (Arthrex, Naples, FL) was placed through the guide, and then a 10-mm reamer was drilled to a depth of 30 mm to create the femoral socket. Arthroscopic inspection of the tunnel in preparation for passage of the graft revealed that the posterior wall had been blown out (**Figure 2**). Soft tissue attached to the posterior cortex of the femoral notch allowed the guide to be displaced too far posteriorly, leading to posterior wall blowout, which compromised 20 mm of the femoral socket and prevented adequate interference screw fixation for the femoral side of the graft.

Discussion

Recognition of the Problem

Although many difficulties may be encountered during graft fixation, techniques have been described for achieving adequate reconstruction.[1] Because an increasing number of orthopaedists perform ACL reconstruction, thorough knowledge of methods to achieve adequate reconstruction despite intraoperative difficulties is essential.

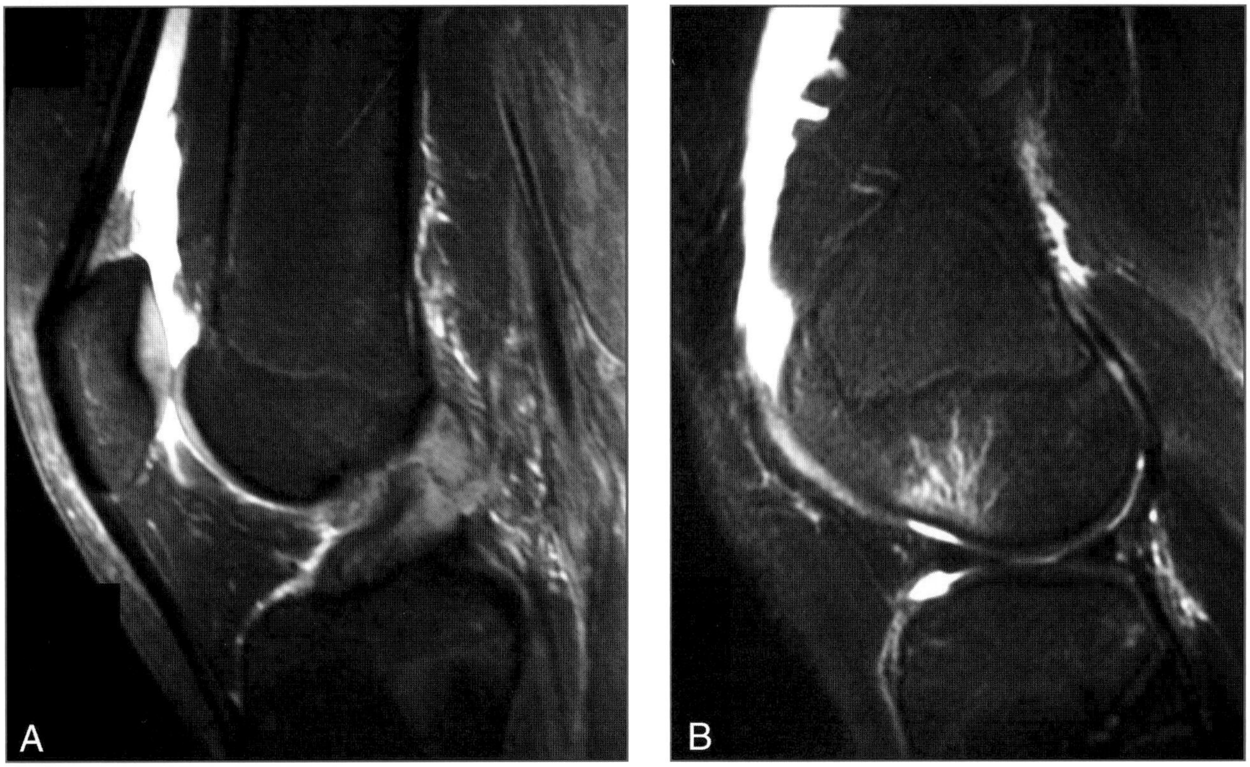

Figure 1 Sagittal T2-weighted MRI scans demonstrating an acute ACL rupture **(A)** and a bone bruise of the lateral femoral condyle at the sulcus terminalis and at the posterior aspect of the lateral tibial plateau **(B)**.

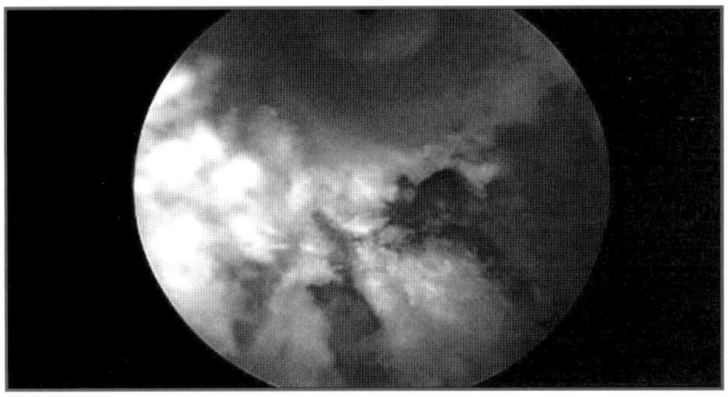

Figure 2 Arthroscopic image of the femoral socket demonstrating a posterior wall blowout. Note the presence of soft tissue only at the posterior portion of the tunnel.

The most common reason for failure of ACL reconstruction and subsequent revision is technical error, which has been implicated as the cause of failure in up to 92% of revisions.[2] The most common error is improper tunnel placement.[1-4] Other technical errors include compromise of bony tunnels, inadequate graft-tunnel interface, improper tensioning of the graft, graft selection errors, inadequate or improper notch preparation, and graft harvest errors.[2,5]

Posterior wall blowout is a complication associated with improper femoral tunnel placement. Improper positioning of either the tibial or femoral tunnel may result in a nonfunctional graft. The femoral tunnel ideally is placed at the 10:30 to 11:00 o'clock position (right knee) and at the 1:00 to 1:30 o'clock position (left knee), with an intact posterior wall of 1 to 2 mm after reaming. The tibial tunnel ideally is placed in the posteromedial footprint of the native ACL in a line congruent with the posterior aspect of the anterior horn of the lateral meniscus, leaving 7 mm of bone anterior to the posterior cruciate ligament (PCL) and 2 mm of bone lateral to the articular surface of the medial tibial plateau after reaming (**Figure 3**). Deviation from these positions may result in a malfunctioning graft.[5]

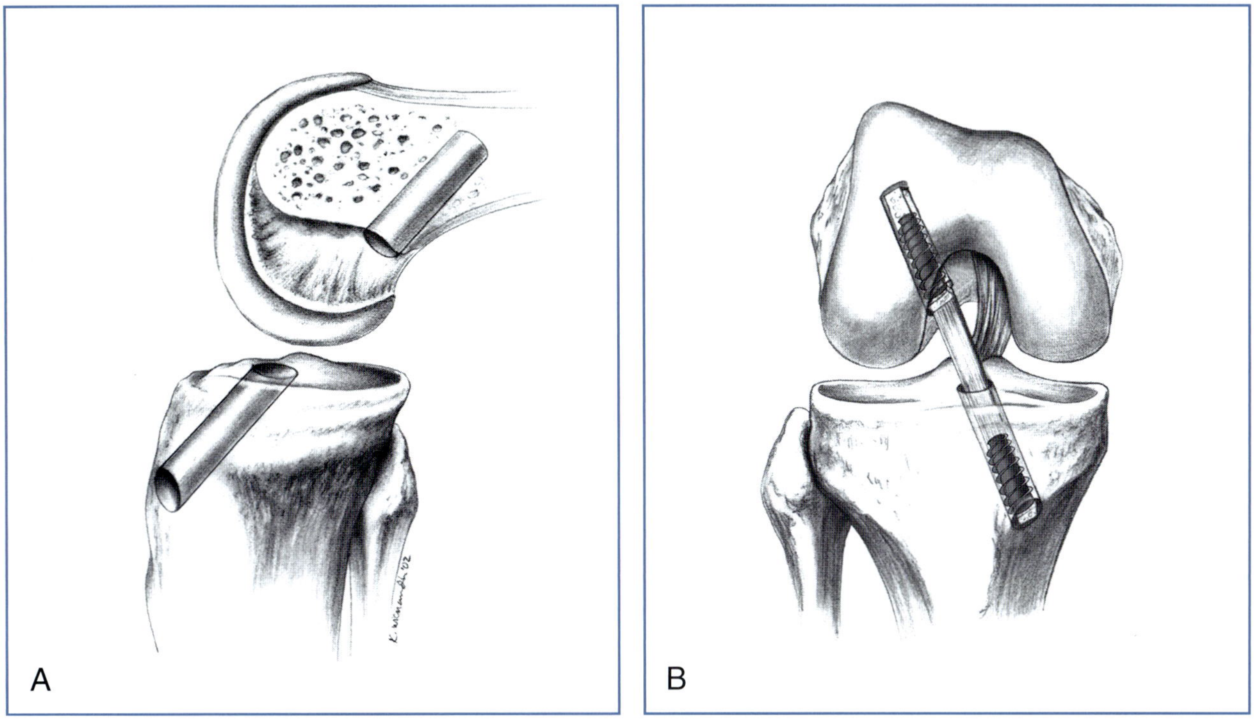

Figure 3 Appropriate ACL tunnel position shown in both sagittal **(A)** and AP **(B)** views. (Reproduced from Bach BR Jr, Fox JA, Mazzocca AD: Revision ACL reconstruction. *Orthopaedic Knowledge Online*. Rosemont, Illinois, American Academy of Orthopaedic Surgeons, 2003.)

Femoral Tunnel Malposition

The femoral tunnel is improperly positioned most frequently.[6] A femoral tunnel that is too anterior will result in a graft that is tight in flexion and lax in extension, whereas a femoral tunnel that is too posterior may result in back wall blowout, which compromises interference screw fixation. A femoral tunnel that is too vertical (12:00 o'clock position) may function in the anteroposterior plane but will manifest rotatory instability, and a femoral tunnel that is too lateral (9:00 or 3:00 o'clock position) will result in graft impingement on the lateral femoral condyle or subsequent excessive notchplasty of the lateral condyle.[7] It is important to recognize malposition intraoperatively and to correct it at the time of initial surgery.

Several steps can minimize the possibility of improper tunnel placement during creation of the femoral socket. First, soft-tissue and bony notchplasties should be performed to remove all soft tissue from the intercondylar notch. This step will allow adequate visualization of the over-the-top position. Soft tissue that remains attached to the posterior cortex of the femur can displace an over-the-top guide to a posterior position. After the guide pin is inserted into the femur, an endoscopic footprint should be established with the appropriately sized reamer, followed by a thorough evaluation of tunnel placement. This footprint should be both visualized and palpated with the probe to confirm that the posterior wall is intact and that the tunnel is not too far anterior (**Figure 4**). If the tunnel footprint is not properly positioned, it should be redrilled until its position is acceptable. If the position of the femoral tunnel is still incorrect after final reaming, potential solutions include incorporation of new tunnels, use of revision ACL fixation techniques (with overlapping tunnels), or alternative fixation techniques.

Posterior wall blowout may be caused by reaming the femoral tunnel too posteriorly (as in the case presentation) or with inadequate knee flexion during

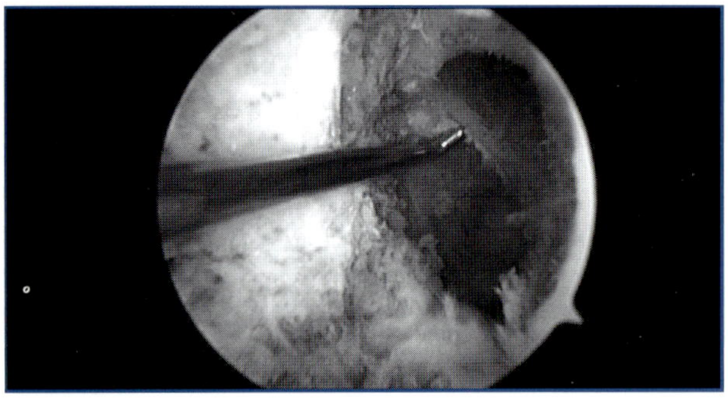

Figure 4 Arthroscopic image demonstrating the femoral socket drilled in the over-the-top position. The posterior wall is visualized and then palpated with a probe to verify that it is only 1- to 2-mm thick to confirm the appropriate intra-articular position.

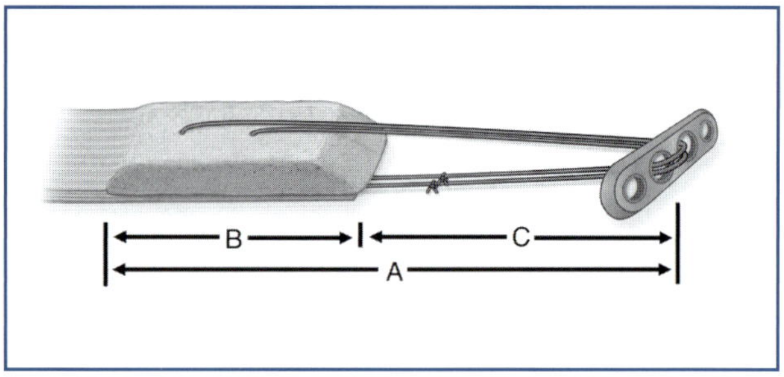

Figure 5 Illustration showing attachment of a patellar tendon bone block to the EndoButton. The total channel length (A) must be measured and the desired depth of graft insertion (B) subtracted to determine the length at which the sutures must be tied (C).

drilling. This problem can be corrected in a number of ways. One option is conversion to a two-incision procedure with direct femoral access for graft fixation; another option, if only a small portion of the posterior wall is blown out, is to use suspension-type fixation, such as the EndoButton (Smith & Nephew Endoscopy, Andover, MA). The bone block from the patellar tendon graft can be attached to the EndoButton using No. 5 nonabsorbable suture (**Figure** 5). Finally, if the blowout is minimal, the graft can be recessed in the femoral socket up to 1 cm, and an interference screw can be used for fixation. However, attempts to salvage a compromised posterior wall may not provide adequate fixation, making conversion to a traditional two-incision technique more prudent.

Conversion to a two-incision technique, as described by Ferrari and associates,[8] allows direct visualization of the femoral fixation, offers multiple options for fixation, and provides a femoral tunnel that does not depend on the tibial tunnel for orientation (**Figure** 6). In this technique, a second skin incision is made in line with the midline of the iliotibial band, extending 4 cm proximal from the lateral femoral epicondyle. The iliotibial band is split in line with its fibers 2 cm anterior to the posterior border, and the vastus lateralis is dissected off the lateral intermuscular septum and femur in a posterior-to-anterior manner. The posterior intercondylar notch is then palpated with blunt dissection and periosteal elevation, with care taken to avoid violating the lateral collateral ligament (LCL) origin (flare of the metaphysis). Bleeding from the lateral geniculate artery must be controlled to prevent a hematoma from forming. Following exposure, a J-shaped femoral guide passer is placed into the appropriate femoral position with arthroscopic assistance, and the bullet tip is placed proximal to the origin of the LCL. After appropriate placement is confirmed, the femoral tunnel is drilled and reamed from proximal to distal into the intra-articular portion of the tunnel (**Figure** 7).

An interference screw placed from the femoral cortex distally may be used to fix the femoral portion of the graft if there is adequate posterior femoral cortex (**Figure** 8). If the femoral cortex has been compromised, even proximally based interference screw fixation may cause the graft to be extruded posteriorly or may further compromise the posterior wall. Fixation with sutures tied over a femoral screw-and-washer construct, with staples, or with a combination of these techniques can be considered.

If an endoscopic footprint is made prior to reaming the entire femoral socket, a malpositioned femoral tunnel can be adjusted without compromising fixation. However, if a complete femoral socket is drilled and later determined to be inappropriately placed, an appropriately placed femoral socket should be drilled. The resulting tunnel overlap is then addressed as it would be during revision ACL reconstruction. This procedure is further detailed in chapter 7. Treatment may include bone grafting the errant femoral tunnel or placing stacked interference screws.

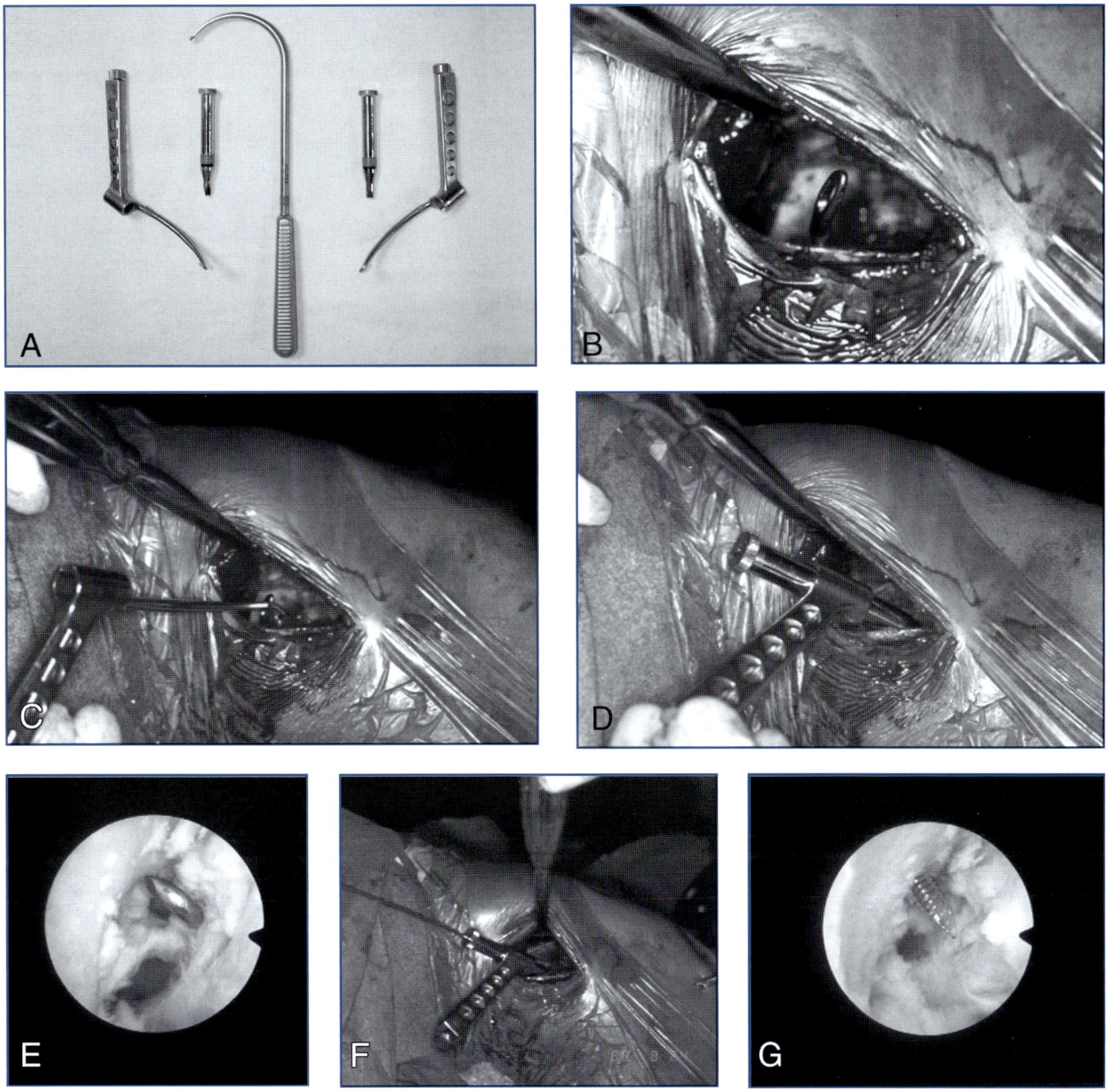

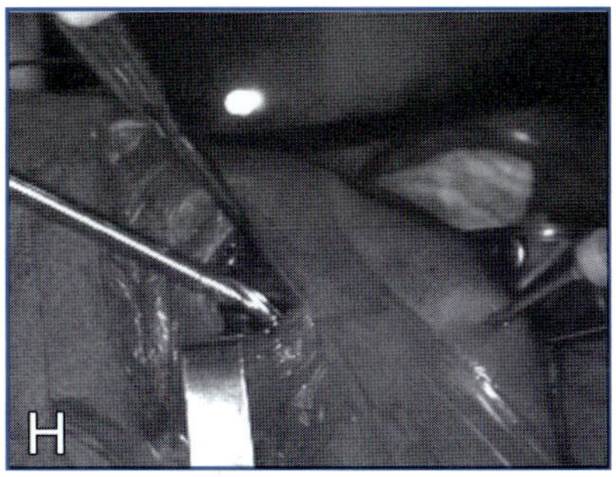

Figure 6 **A,** Rear-entry instruments for two-incision ACL reconstruction (Acufex, Smith & Nephrew, Andover, MA) Intraoperative photographs showing use of rear-entry instruments for two-incision ACL reconstruction. **B,** The J-shaped femoral guide passer is placed through the anteromedial portal, through the intercondylar notch, and out the lateral incision. **C,** The tip of the rear entry guide is placed in the J-shaped suture passer to bring the guide intra-articularly into the intercondylar notch. **D,** Once the guide is place, the bullet is placed in the guide in preparation for placing the pin. **E,** Arthroscopic image showing the rear-entry guide in the over-the-top position. **F,** The guide pin is drilled. **G,** Arthroscopic image showing the guide pin in place. **H,** A 10-mm reamer is advanced over the guide pin.

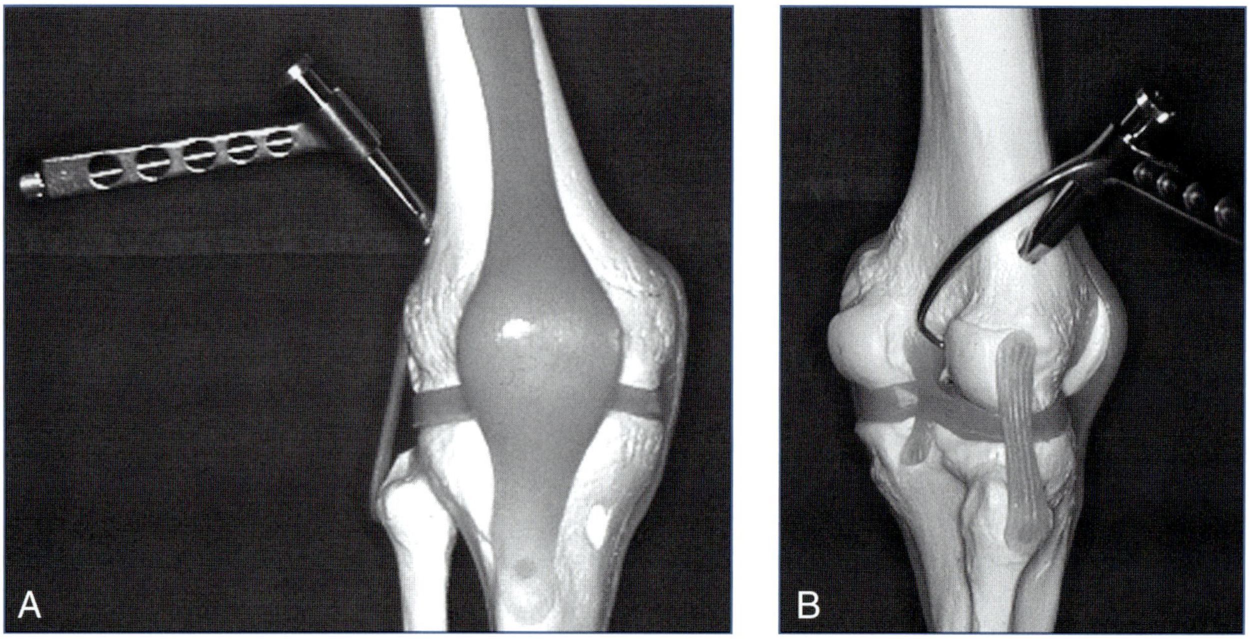

Figure 7 **A,** Use of a rear-entry femoral guide. Note that the bullet tip is placed at the flare of the metaphysis. **B,** The intra-articular position of the rear-entry guide in the over-the-top position. (Reproduced with permission from Ferrari J, Bush-Joseph C, Bach B: Anterior cruciate ligament reconstruction using bone-patellar tendon-bone grafts: Autograft and allograft endoscopic techniques and two-incision autograft technique. *Oper Tech Sports Med* 1999;7:156-171.)

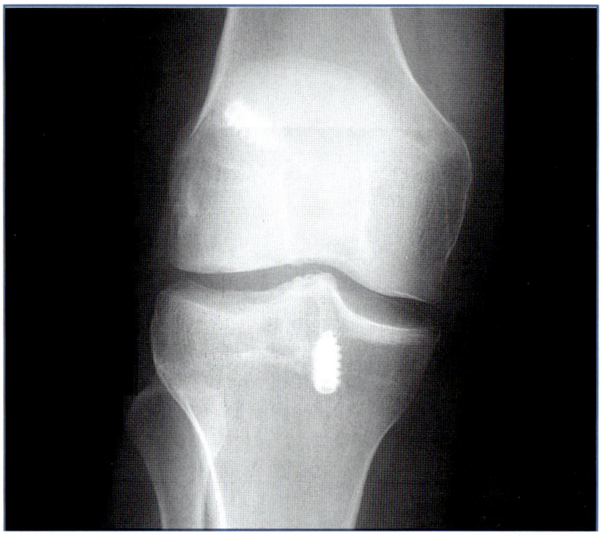

Figure 8 AP radiograph showing a femoral interference screw placed on the lateral femoral cortex from a two-incision technique.

Tibial Tunnel Malposition

An improperly placed tibial tunnel also will result in a predictably poor ACL reconstruction; however, appropriate placement of a tibial tunnel is somewhat more variable. Appropriate placement of the tibial tunnel is in the posteromedial footprint of the ACL stump, approximately 7 mm anterior to the PCL fibers in the center of the intercondylar notch. If viewed on a lateral radiograph, the tibial tunnel should be parallel and just posterior to a line congruent with Blumensaat's lines (Figure 3, *A*).

Graft fixation in a tibial tunnel that is too far anterior will result in impingement in extension and excessive tension in flexion. Reaming a tibial tunnel significantly too far anterior may compromise the anterior tibial wall. A graft fixed too posterior will impinge on the PCL, and a tunnel reamed too far posterior may compromise the PCL attachment. A graft fixed too medial or lateral will impinge on its respective condylar wall or will cause the surgeon to perform an excessive notchplasty to prevent impingement.

If the tibial tunnel is reamed slightly anterior, it may be possible to (1) rotate the BTB graft so that the graft's tendinous portion faces posteriorly or (2) enlarge the tunnel with a burr and use a larger interference screw to push the graft to a more posterior position. A tibial tunnel that is too far posterior may be improved by placing the cancellous portion of the BTB graft or an interference screw posterior to the graft; this step will help place the graft in a more anterior position in the tunnel.

If anterior cortical disruption has occurred, methods other than interference screw fixation should be considered. In this situation, the fixation may cause the graft to extrude through the compromised anterior cortex. As with posterior wall blowout, suture over a screw-and-washer construct or staple fixation may be more appropriate with intraoperative revision of the tibial tunnel or anterior wall blowout. A further consideration is that tibial fixation is relatively subcutaneous compared with distal femoral fixation, and prominent hardware may be more problematic for the patient.

Additional Graft Fixation Problems

Interference screw fixation has been shown to be biomechanically superior to staples, suture fixation, or screw-and-washer fixation.[9] Although bioabsorbable interference screws currently are popular, early biomechanical studies report that they had less pullout strength than their metallic counterparts.[10] The additional complication of screw breakage during insertion of bioabsorbable materials also has been of some concern. Under ideal conditions, interference screws may be the fixation device of choice, but intraoperative circumstances may dictate that alternative forms of fixation may be more advantageous in some patients. Therefore, it is important to become familiar with a variety of fixation options.

If a bone plug is broken during implantation, several salvage options may be available. If the plug is broken in the longitudinal plane, such that its diameter is inadequate to fill the tunnel, cross-pin fixation augmented by bone graft may be used. If the plug is broken transversely, such that the plug is shorter than 15 mm, Krackow sutures may be placed in the soft-tissue portion of the graft and then tied around a screw-and-washer post,[3] as shown in Figure 3, chapter 1.

Difficulty also may arise while placing the interference screw. Ideally, the interference screw will be the same length as the bone plug, and each thread of the screw will be in contact with the bone block and the tunnel. The relationship of the screw to the bone plug needs to be evaluated intraoperatively because screw malposition may result in early failure. If the screw is distal to the bone plug, it may be advanced inadequately, resulting in decreased pullout strength. The screw also may be advanced too proximally, causing a decreased screw-bone plug interface that requires reevaluation of the graft because the head of the screw may damage the tendinous portion of the graft. A divergent relationship between the screw and bone plug (especially greater than 15°) also will cause a decreased screw-bone plug interface.

If the screw-bone plug interface is appropriately matched in length and fixation is still inadequate, the bone plug-tunnel gap should be evaluated. If the gap is 1 to 2 mm, a 7- or 8-mm interference screw should provide adequate fixation in younger patients. However, more ACL reconstructions are performed in older patients who may have poor bone quality. Thus, a 9-mm interference screw may be necessary, even for 1- to 2-mm gaps. As the gap increases to 3 to 4 mm, it may be prudent to use a 9-mm or larger interference screw based on bone quality. With continued concern about fixation strength, the addition of suture tied over a screw-and-washer construct will provide additional pullout strength.

Graft-Construct Mismatch

Tunnel-graft length mismatch is another type of fixation difficulty encountered intraoperatively with patellar tendon grafts. A graft may be too long or too short for methods of planned fixation. Identifying excessively long BTB grafts before tunnel placement may allow the position of the tunnels to be adjusted to accommodate a longer tibial tunnel (60°or 65°) and ultimately a longer graft. This angle can be quantified using the N + 7 rule,[11] in which N is the length of the tendinous portion of the graft and N + 7 is the angle in degrees used on the tibial guide.

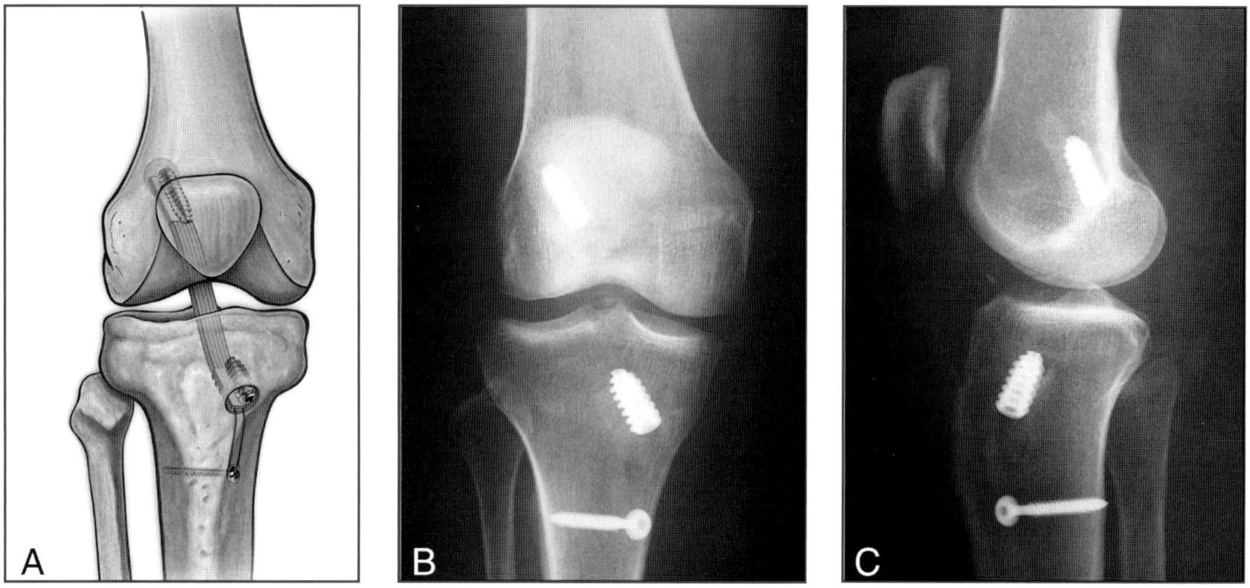

Figure 9 **A,** A free bone block for graft-construct mismatch in which the sutures in the graft are tied over a fixation post. AP **(B)** and lateral **(C)** radiographs show the addition of a patellar tendon autograft fixed with a free bone block technique.

If the graft is still excessively long, despite more vertical placement of the tunnels, or if it is recognized after placement of tunnels, several techniques may be used to achieve appropriate graft tension. If the graft is excessively long, as in the case of undiagnosed patella alta, the femoral bone plug may be completely flipped to overlap the proximal portion of the tendon and then fixed with standard interference techniques. Typically, however, there will not be enough excess graft for this solution, and another technique will be necessary to achieve appropriate graft tension.

Small amounts of mismatch can be accommodated by recession of the graft in the femoral tunnel (up to 10 mm) or by shortening the tibial bone plug. Another technique involves rotating the graft up to 540° to shorten the tendon without compromising mechanical strength.[8] Our preferred technique involves creating a free bone block, which requires carefully removing the bone plug from the tibial portion of the graft and placing a Krackow suture in the soft-tissue portion of the graft. After the graft is fixed on the femoral side, the Krackow sutures are tensioned, the free bone block is advanced in the tibial tunnel, and a metal interference screw is placed over the bone block (**Figure 9**, *A*). The soft-tissue suture is then sutured over a post to provide back-up fixation (**Figure 9**, *B* and *C*).

Inadequate patellar tendon length, such as in patella baja, ideally is identified on preoperative imaging studies, which enables the surgeon to have a more informed discussion with the patient regarding graft selection. If, intraoperatively, the length of the tendinous portion of the graft is found to be inadequate, the graft may be converted to a single bone plug-tendon construct after sharply dissecting off the tendinous portion of the distal bone plug from the bone and using soft-tissue fixation techniques on the tibia. If these conditions are not recognized preoperatively, harvested graft from patients with Osgood-Schlatter disease or, more rarely, Sinding-Larsen-Johansson disease may mimic graft from patients with patella baja. In these instances, the surgeon initially may think there is inadequate tendon length. On further examination, the surgeon will observe accessory ossification of either the tibial (Osgood-Schlatter) or patellar portion (Sinding-Larsen-Johansson) of the graft, which can be corrected by curettage of the excess bone, resulting in normal tendon length with acceptable bone plugs.

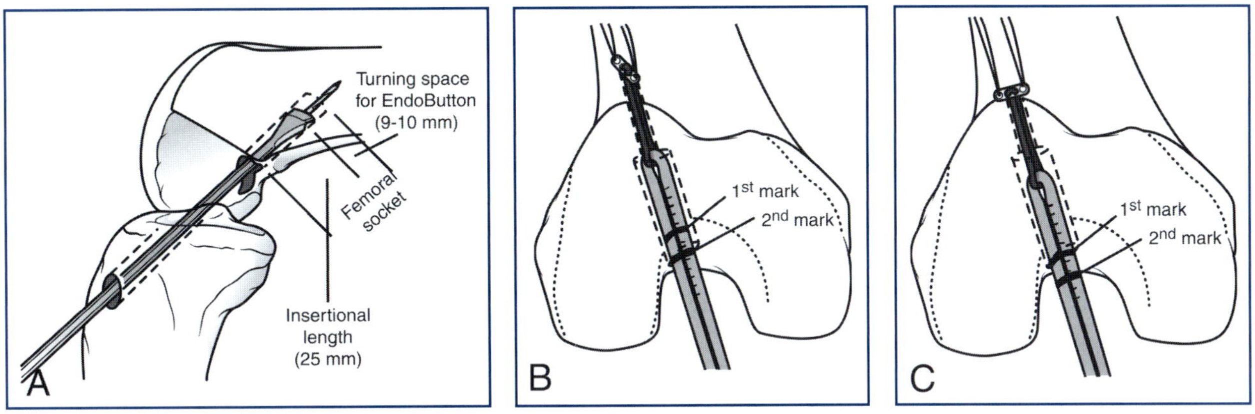

Figure 10 **A,** Femoral socket drilling for EndoButton insertion. The femoral socket must be drilled 10 mm longer than the desired graft insertion length to allow the EndoButton to flip on the lateral cortex. **B,** The hamstrings graft is inserted 10 mm beyond the desired insertion depth to allow the EndoButton to flip outside the femoral cortex. **C,** The graft is positioned at the final insertion depth with the EndoButton locked on the femoral cortex.

Complications of Hamstrings Fixation

Although techniques to correct intraoperative difficulties using hamstrings graft may be extrapolated from those used in patellar tendon reconstruction, differences in technique must be considered. Each type of soft-tissue fixation for hamstrings grafts may have unique complications. For example, hamstrings tendon fixation with staples may result in graft necrosis or amputation and early failure. Salvage techniques include use of suture tied over screw and washer to supplement interference screw fixation, as well as other soft-tissue fixation techniques. Another method of femoral fixation used in hamstrings-ACL reconstruction is suspension-type fixation, such as the EndoButton CL.

Femoral tunnel preparation for EndoButton fixation is similar to that used in patellar tendon reconstruction, except that the femoral tunnel is reamed 10 mm longer than the desired graft-tunnel interface to allow the EndoButton to flip in the soft tissue outside of the 4.5-mm proximal femoral aperture[12] (**Figure 10**). A length of synthetic continuous loop appropriate to incorporate at least 20 mm of graft in the femoral tunnel is chosen. A lead suture is used to pull the EndoButton through the femoral tunnel. After advancement through the tunnel, tension on the trailing suture allows the EndoButton to toggle on the femoral cortex. The graft is then tensioned and subsequently fixed distally. This suspension-type fixation is adequate with grafts of different lengths because the synthetic continuous loop is available in multiple lengths, allowing incorporation of both shorter and longer grafts.

Difficulties associated with the EndoButton are somewhat distinct from those of standard patellar tendon fixation techniques.[13] If the standard-diameter reamer (usually 7 to 10 mm) inadvertently reams too deep and the femoral cortex is violated, the EndoButton cannot be used for proximal fixation[10] because the device is only 12 mm long; violation of the femoral cortex may allow the device to disengage from the cortex. Salvage techniques for this situation include use of a bioabsorbable interference screw for femoral socket fixation or cross-pin fixation through the graft. In addition, the femoral tunnel can be exposed from the lateral cortex, and a screw and washer can be used for soft-tissue fixation.

A second difficulty occurs when the EndoButton is pulled into but does not flip within the soft tissues outside the femur or if an attempt is made to flip the EndoButton within the 4.5-mm tunnel. These problems will prevent the EndoButton from locking on the femur, and the graft will pull distally through the tunnel when tensioned. If the placement or stability of the EndoButton is uncertain, intraoperative fluoroscopy may confirm its position on the femoral cortex. A safety stitch placed in the trail portion of the EndoButton can help to disengage it for repeat passage or graft removal.

The hamstrings graft-tunnel gap is more difficult to correct than patellar tendon grafts in which a bone plug-tunnel gap may be corrected with larger interference screws. Significant gapping may result in a windshield wiper effect, enlarging the femoral tunnel and contributing to instability. Careful preparation is the most effective way to avoid this pitfall, but if it exists, the gap may be filled by incorporating bone graft within the individual strands of the tendon graft. If bioabsorbable screws are used for soft-tissue graft fixation, a more gradual postoperative rehabilitation protocol should be considered because of decreased fixation strength, particularly in tibial fixation.

Management and Outcome Summary

The patient described in the case study had 20 mm of posterior wall blowout, preventing adequate interference screw fixation in the tunnel. We believed that endoscopic interference screw fixation might not be adequate and that there was not appropriate bony contact for enough of the graft. Because of our concerns about the stability of graft fixation, we converted to a two-incision technique, allowing direct access to femoral fixation. A new divergent tunnel was drilled from the lateral cortex of the femur (**Figure 11**). The graft was then passed and fixed on the femoral side with an interference screw at the lateral cortex of the femur, resulting in excellent fixation. Routine postoperative rehabilitation followed, and the patient had an uneventful postoperative course, with return to sports at 6 months postoperatively.

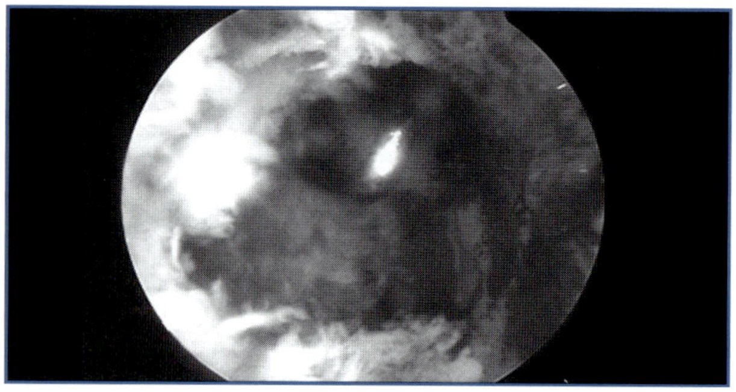

Figure 11 Arthroscopic image showing the rear-entry guide at the intra-articular site of the new femoral socket. The tunnel will be divergent from the endoscopic tunnel that was drilled.

Strategies to Minimize Common Complications

Graft fixation problems during ACL reconstruction usually can be avoided by careful attention to surgical technique. Strict attention to tunnel position is crucial and should be checked periodically during tunnel reaming. Adequate visualization of the over-the-top position is critical before reaming the femoral socket; the position also must be verified after the footprint is established. Because graft fixation problems occasionally occur, all the instruments that may be required must be available in the operating room, specifically a rear-entry ACL guide for a two-incision technique and a multitude of fixation options, such as metal and bioabsorbable screws and screw-and-post fixation. Having several alternative fixation options available will allow adequate graft fixation for nearly any problem encountered.

References

1. Cain E, Gillogly S, Andrews J: Management of intraoperative complications associated with autogenous patellar tendon graft anterior cruciate ligament reconstruction. *Instr Course Lect* 2003;52:359-367.
2. Wetzler M, Getelman M, Friedman M, Bartolozzi A: Revision anterior cruciate ligament surgery: Etiology of failures. *Oper Tech Sports Med* 1998;6:64-70.
3. Dalton J, Harner C: Surgical techniques to correct nonanatomic femoral tunnels. *Oper Tech Sports Med* 1998;6:83-90.
4. Phillips B, Haynes D:. Complications of anterior cruci-

ate ligament reconstruction. *Instr Course Lect* 2002;51:329-333.

5. Azar F: Revision anterior cruciate ligament reconstruction. *Instr Course Lect* 2002;51:335-342.
6. Harner CD, Griffin JR, Dunteman RC, Annunziata CC, Friedman MJ: Evaluation and treatment of recurrent instability after anterior cruciate ligament reconstruction. *Instr Course Lect* 2001;50:463-474.
7. Johnson DL, Miller MD, Fu FH: The arthroscopic "impingement test" during anterior cruciate ligament reconstruction. *Arthroscopy* 1993;9:714-717.
8. Ferrari J, Bush-Joseph C, Bach B: Anterior cruciate ligament reconstruction using bone-patellar tendon-bone grafts: Autograft and allograft endoscopic techniques and two-incision autograft technique. *Oper Tech Sports Med* 1999;7:156-171.
9. Kurosaka M, Yoshiya S, Andrish J: A biomechanical comparison of different surgical techniques in graft fixation in anterior cruciate ligament reconstruction. *Am J Sports Med* 1987;15:225-229.
10. Pena F, Grontvedt T, Brown G, Aune A, Engebretsen L: Comparison of failure strength between metallic and absorbable interference screws. *Am J Sports Med* 1996;24:329-334.
11. Miller M, Hinkin D: The "N + 7 rule" for tibial tunnel placement in endoscopic anterior cruciate ligament reconstruction. *Arthroscopy* 1996;15:124-126.
12. Graf B, Davies W: Endobutton fixation of hamstring tendon grafts. *Oper Tech Sports Med* 1999;7:189-194.
13. Lyons PM, Graf BK: Pearls and pitfalls of Endobutton fixation. *Tech Orthop* 1998;13:299-305.

Chapter 3

Extensor Mechanism Compromise and Patellar Fracture

Randall J. Risinger, MD
Bernard R. Bach, Jr, MD

Case Presentation

History

A 26-year-old basketball player felt an immediate pop after a twisting hyperflexion injury to his left knee but attempted to continue playing. After a second pivoting injury during the same game, he stopped playing because he could not fully extend his knee. Subsequently, a large effusion developed, and he presented to the emergency department for examination. Radiographs obtained at that time ruled out a periarticular fracture. The patient presented for specialty evaluation 5 days after the injury.

At initial presentation, the patient held his knee flexed 10° and described pain with further extension. Physical examination revealed that the extensor mechanism was intact, and the patellar examination was unremarkable. There was a 1+ effusion and lateral joint tenderness, knee range of motion was 10° to 100°, the posterior drawer test was negative, varus/valgus stress testing at 30° was normal, the Lachman test was a low grade III with a soft end point, an attempt at pivot-shift testing produced guarding, and the dial test was negative at 30° and 90°. KT-1000 arthrometer (MEDmetric Corp, San Diego, CA) testing revealed a 9-mm side-to-side maximum manual difference.

The knee radiographs were normal. MRI revealed an effusion, anterior cruciate ligament (ACL) disruption with classic lateral compartment bone bruises, and a bucket-handle lateral meniscus tear displaced into the intercondylar notch (**Figure 1**).

The patient was counseled about treatment options for his ACL injury. Based on his desire to continue sports participation for more than 6 hours per week in activities that would put his knee at risk for further pivoting episodes and a high (> 6 mm) KT-1000 side-to-side difference, ACL reconstruction was recommended. Initial meniscal surgery to assist with motion recovery and staged ACL reconstruction also were discussed. However, the patient wished to proceed with a single-stage reconstruction procedure; he had professional time constraints and was concerned about insurance coverage during an upcoming job transition.

By 12 days after the injury, gains in his range of motion were significant; he lacked only 2° of terminal extension and was able to flex beyond 125°. Because of this rapid improvement, a single-stage procedure was selected. After a

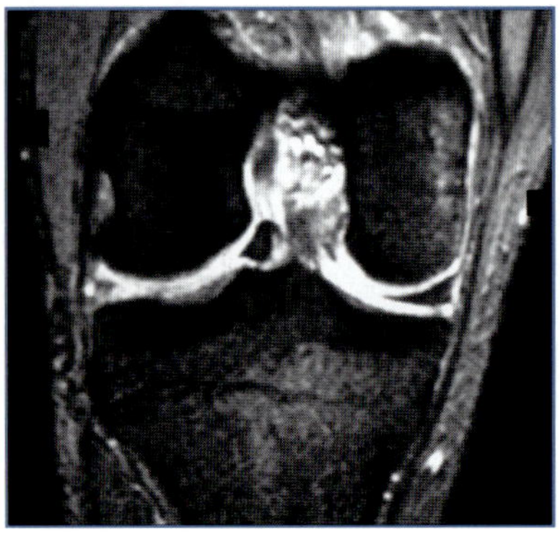

Figure 1 Coronal MRI scan showing a bucket-handle lateral meniscus tear displaced into the intercondylar notch.

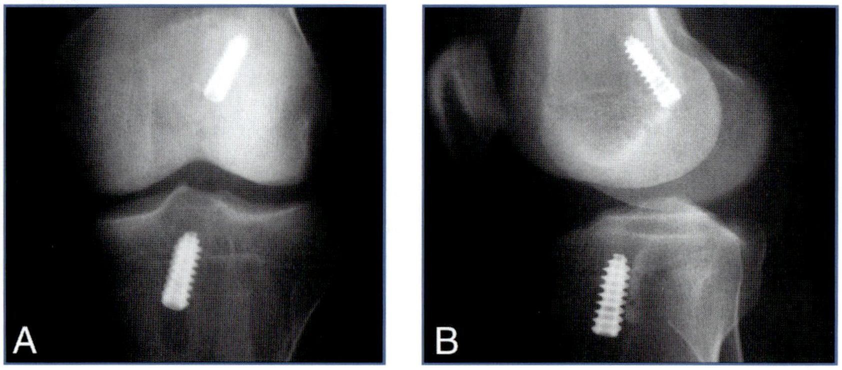

Figure 2 Initial postoperative AP **(A)** and lateral **(B)** radiographs following ACL reconstruction.

complete discussion about graft alternatives, patellar tendon autograft was chosen.

The patient underwent an uncomplicated arthroscopically assisted ACL reconstruction and lateral meniscus repair 21 days after the injury. A standard single-incision endoscopic reconstruction technique[1] was used, and an inside-out meniscus repair was performed using an accessory incision. Diagnostic arthroscopy did not reveal any other significant intra-articular pathology.

The patient was discharged home from the recovery room after physical therapy instruction, and his initial postoperative recovery was uneventful. Radiographs obtained on postoperative day 8 revealed appropriate tunnel and interference screw positions (**Figure 2**). The patient had complete hyperextension and flexion to 90°, and his rehabilitation was progressing uneventfully.

He was instructed to wear a brace for the first 6 weeks postoperatively to protect his extensor mechanism. He was allowed weight bearing as tolerated with the brace locked in full extension for the first 2 weeks, and then allowed to unlock the brace for ambulation. He was allowed immediate full motion without the brace when not weight bearing.

Current Problem and Treatment

Five weeks postoperatively, the patient fell and sustained a direct blow to the patella. He was not wearing the brace at the time and admitted to brace noncompliance. A large effusion developed immediately, and he presented for examination.

Physical examination revealed a 30° extension lag and significant pain with quadriceps activation. Radiographs showed a displaced transverse patellar fracture at the level of the proximal harvest bed (**Figure 3**).

The patient subsequently required urgent open reduction and internal fixation with two partially threaded cannulated screws and a tension band construct (**Figure 4**).

Discussion

Recognizing the Problem and Situations at Risk

ACL injury is extremely common, especially in the athletic population. It is estimated that 100,000 new ACL injuries occur annually, and one of every 3,000 people will sustain an ACL injury in a given year.2 In the past, these injuries often would preclude return to high-level sports activities. With current surgical techniques for ACL reconstruction, knee stability can be restored, and injured athletes can return to strenuous activities more than 90% of the time, usually within 6 months. Given this success rate, individuals wishing to return to demanding activities are often candidates for ACL reconstruction. When counseling these patients, however, it is important to communicate potential adverse outcomes of ACL reconstruction.

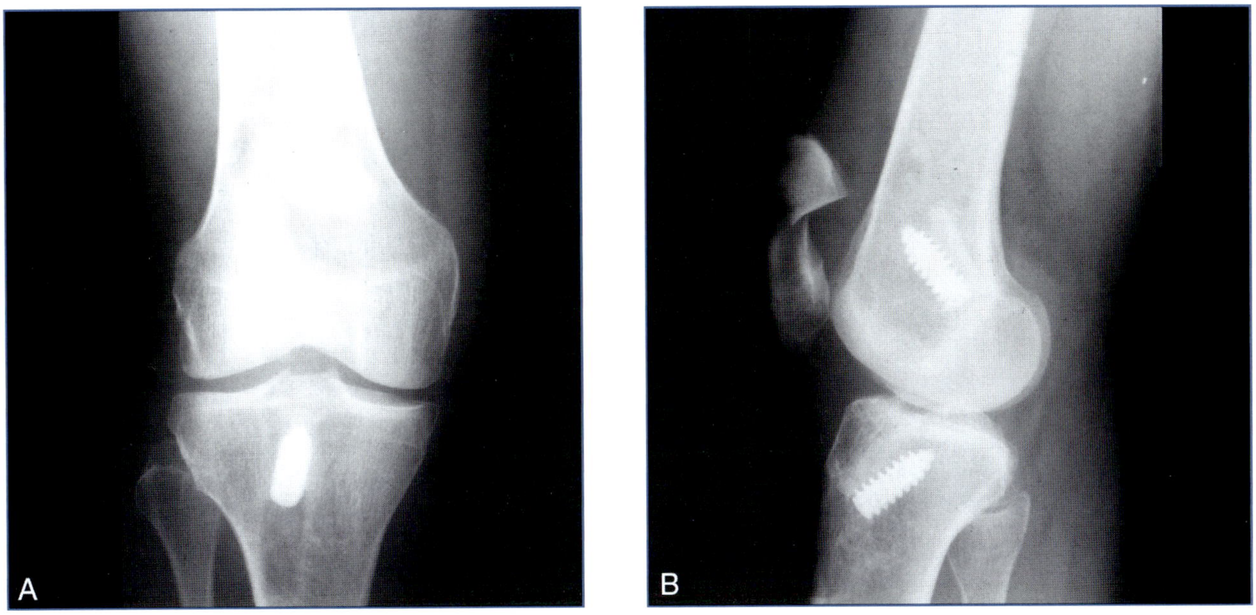

Figure 3 AP **(A)** and lateral **(B)** radiographs show a postoperative transverse patellar fracture. (Reproduced from Carpenter JE, Kasman R, Matthews LS: Fractures of the patella. *Instr Course Lect* 1994;43:97-108.)

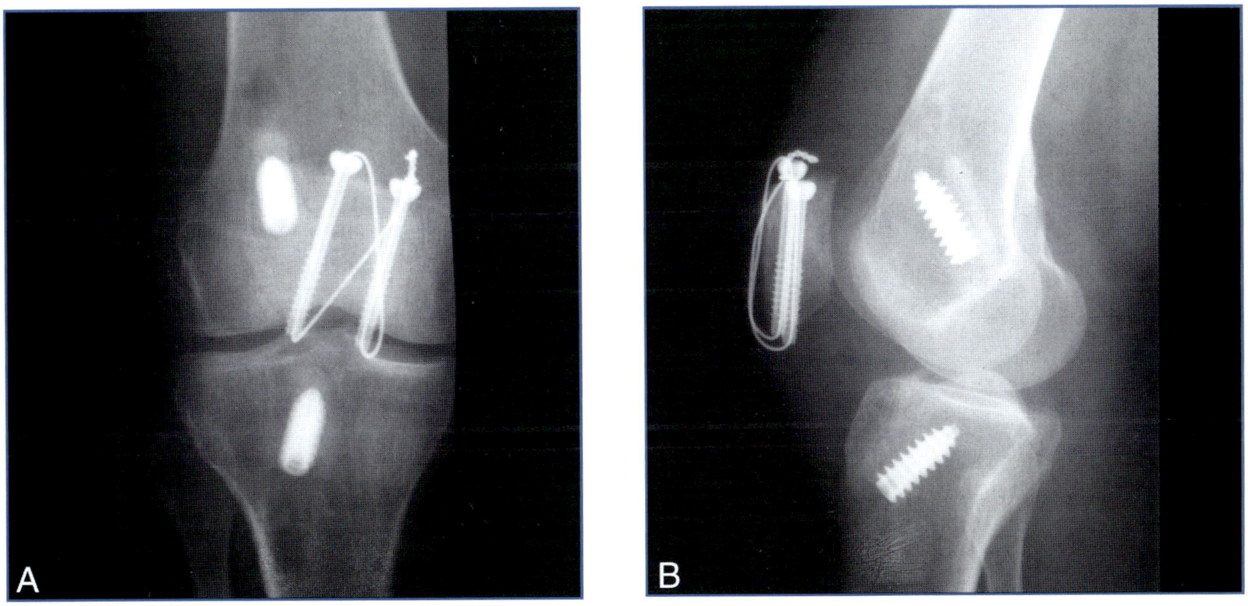

Figure 4 Postoperative AP **(A)** and lateral **(B)** radiographs showing anatomic fracture reduction and cannulated screw/tension band construct. (Reproduced from Carpenter JE, Kasman R, Matthews LS: Fractures of the patella. *Instr Course Lect* 1994;43:97-108.)

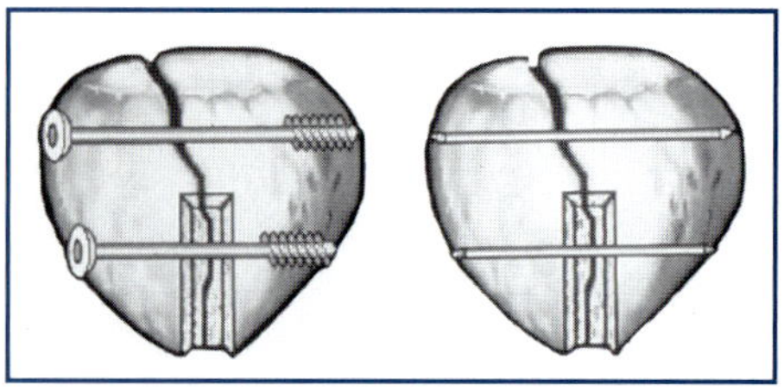

Figure 5 Longitudinal patellar fractures may be fixed with transverse screws (left) or K-wires (right). (Reproduced from Cain EL Jr, Gillogl SD, Andrews JR: Management of intraoperative complications associated with autogenous patellar tendon graft anterior cruciate ligament reconstruction. *Instr Course Lect* 2003;52:359-367.)

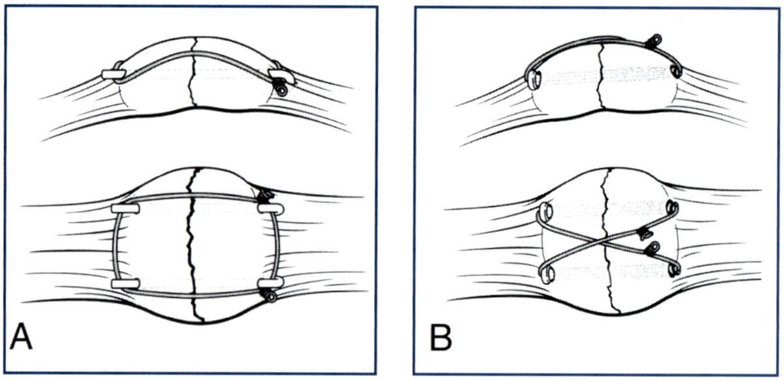

Figure 6 Fracture fixation can be accomplished with a tension band/K-wire construct **(A)** or with cannulated screws and tension wires **(B)**. (Reproduced from Carpenter JE, Kasman R, Matthews LS: Fractures of the patella. *Instr Course Lect* 1994;43:97-108.)

Complications specific to the extensor mechanism are among the most common, and this chapter illustrates their causes, prevention, and proper treatment.

Unusual macrotraumatic extensor mechanism complications occur specifically after harvest of the central-third patellar tendon (intraoperative or postoperative patellar fracture and patellar tendon rupture) and are related to both harvest technique and, possibly, postoperative management. However, anterior knee pain is the most common problem that may affect the clinical outcome of ACL reconstruction and, although pain is more common after patellar tendon harvest, it also occurs following hamstrings-ACL reconstruction. A meta-analysis of ACL reconstructions revealed a 17% incidence of anterior knee pain with use of autologous patellar tendon and a 12% incidence with use of autologous hamstrings tendon.[3] Buss and assocciates[4] reported a 22% incidence of anterior knee pain in ACL-deficient patients who did not undergo reconstruction. Thus, multiple factors, in addition to the type of graft used for ACL reconstruction, clearly contribute to anterior knee pain in these patients. In fact, several authors have reported that anterior knee pain is closely associated with postoperative loss of terminal extension, regardless of the type of graft selected.[5]

Patellar fractures are unusual after patellar autograft procedures, with a reported prevalence of less than 1%.[6] Bone block removal creates an inherent stress riser at the junction of the graft bed corners and the remaining patella. These fractures can occur either intraoperatively or postoperatively. Intraoperative fractures are less common, are usually longitudinal and nondisplaced, and occur during patellar bone block removal. Postoperative fractures typically are displaced stellate or transverse fractures that disrupt the extensor mechanism. The latter commonly result from direct trauma during brace noncompliance or from increased tensile stresses during aggressive rehabilitation.[7] However, if postoperative weight bearing or range of motion is limited excessively, secondary osteopenia also could place patients at risk for subsequent fracture.

Management of Patellar Fractures

Management of an intraoperative patellar fracture relies on recognition of the fracture followed by appropriate fixation. Longitudinal fractures may be repaired using transverse lag screws or Kirschner wires (K-wires) (**Figure 5**). Transverse fractures are repaired using lag screws and/or a tension band wire technique (**Figure 6**), as illustrated in the case study. Postoperative patellar fractures are managed similarly. Rehabilitation following fracture fixation warrants immediate gentle range of motion and weight bearing in extension. A hinged knee brace is used to control knee motion and prevent loss of fixation until radiographic healing is confirmed.

Viola and Vianello[8] reported three displaced transverse patellar fractures in a series of 1,320 ACL reconstructions with patellar autograft. These fractures occurred between 8 and 12 weeks postoperatively and were treated with open reduction and internal fixation with subsequent hardware removal. At final follow-up, this complication did not affect the long-term clinical outcome. Other studies confirm that early recognition and internal fixation allow adequate rehabilitation without compromising the final clinical outcome.[9]

Preventing Patellar Fractures

We believe that proper graft harvesting techniques are essential to minimize the risk of a patellar fracture, which usually is the result of an overaggressive bone plug harvest in a patient with a small, hypoplastic patella. The surgeon should be aware of this potential risk whenever an osteotome is used to lever a bone plug that has not been cut adequately. In fashioning the patellar bone plug, the cortex is scored with an oscillating saw, and an equilateral triangle is made on profile with the saw to avoid penetrating the articular cartilage; the blade is angled approximately 30° centrally, and the final blade depth should not exceed 6 to 7 mm (**Figure 7**). When making the proximal crosscut, the saw blade is held at 45° to the cortex to avoid overshooting the sagittal cuts. Excessively long or deep cuts may create a stress riser that could lead to fracture. We use a curved 3/8-inch osteotome to gently remove a trapezoidal profile graft while ensuring that we do not lever it from the osseous bed.

Cadaveric studies of the residual bone plug defect geometry (eg, trapezoidal or cylindric) have shown that patellae with round-cornered or cylindric defects are more resistant to fracture during impact loading[10,11] but not during tensile loading.[12] We do not know of any clinical studies that relate bone plug geometry to fracture risk, and we do not use cylindric saws or create tapered cuts on the patella.

Primary bone grafting of the harvest site with autograft from canal reamings is recommended, especially if the patellar bone block is wider than 10 mm or deeper than 6 mm.[13] Tsuda and associates[14] reported a significant reduction in patellar pain symptoms at an average of 35 months postoperatively when grafting produced a residual patellar defect less than 2 mm deep. The statistical power necessary to prove that grafting significantly reduces

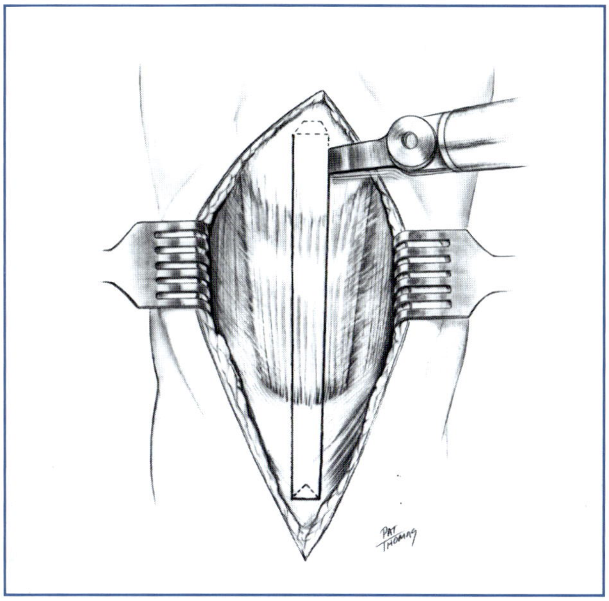

Figure 7 The graft is harvested with an oscillating saw. The patellar plug is trapezoidal on profile. (Reproduced with permission from Hardin GT, Bach BR Jr, Bush-Joseph CA, et al: Endoscopic single incision ACL reconstruction using patellar tendon autograft: Surgical technique. *J Knee Surg* 2003;16:135-147.)

the possibility of postoperative fracture virtually precludes performing such a study; however, it makes sense intuitively.

Contemporary postoperative rehabilitation programs emphasize patellar mobilization and immediate full passive extension combined with night extension bracing. Early active range of motion, straight leg raises, closed chain exercises, and immediate weight bearing in extension are allowed to promote early muscle control and quadriceps reactivation. Brace protection during weight bearing is recommended for 6 weeks after harvest of the patellar tendon to minimize the chance of patellar fracture.

Management of Patellar Tendon Rupture

Patellar tendon rupture is another unusual complication following central-third harvest. We are aware of only 11 instances reported in the English language orthopaedic literature; however, this complication likely is underreported. Of these 11 instances, nine occurred within 10 months after the index procedure. The other two occurred at 3 and 6 years after graft harvest.[15] Three ruptures occurred at the tibial insertion; eight involved proximal avulsions, and six of the eight occurred after a Marshall-MacIntosh procedure. This procedure requires a large portion of the prepatellar retinaculum in continuity with the central-third patellar tendon, and it is postulated that direct damage to, or devascularization of, the remaining tendon may be causally related. However, these speculative etiologies have not been proved, given the large number of Marshall-MacIntosh procedures performed without subsequent patellar tendon rupture. In 10 of the 11 ruptures, some form of trauma could be identified (eg, direct impact, hyperflexion, or forceful quadriceps muscle contraction). No related trauma could be identified in the remaining rupture.[15]

Devascularization, an alteration in tendon healing and remodeling, or injury to the remaining tendon at the time of graft harvest or defect closure are believed to be possible causes of patellar tendon rupture when contemporary harvesting techniques are used. Either proximal focal tendon necrosis caused by excessive tension during closure or iatrogenic tendon shortening and secondary increased insertional shear force may lead to rupture associated with defect closure. However, among the ruptures described, only three defects had been closed, two had not been reapproximated, and closure or otherwise was not identified for the remaining six. Thus, whether closure of the defect increases the risk of rupture is unclear. We prefer to loosely close the defect with the knee flexed at 70° and subsequently close the paratenon over the tendon.

In principle, the remaining two thirds of the patellar tendon should be strong enough to withstand rupture during quadriceps muscle contraction; general consensus is that a tendon must be compromised by 50% before it will fail under significant loads and by 75% before rupture occurs under physiologic loads.[16] Clinically, this appears to be true because patellar tendon ruptures are unusual after harvest of the central third. We have observed that the affected patellar tendon frequently is 20% to 30% wider postoperatively than the contralateral tendon. We cannot recollect any patient in whom the actual tendon, despite harvest, was in fact narrower than the unaffected contralateral tendon by 3 months postoperatively.

Early recognition of a postoperative patellar tendon rupture allows primary suture repair through bone holes, either proximally or distally. This repair technique is commonly reinforced with a temporary McLaughlin-type wire with good results. Autograft or allograft tissue supplementation has not been used extensively. Postoperative rehabilitation includes immediate gentle passive range of motion and protected weight bearing in extension. Initially, 45° of flexion usually is allowed, but it also is based on an intraoperative assessment of the tension and stability of the repair during passive flexion. Range of motion begins slowly at 4 weeks postoperatively, active knee extension begins at 8 weeks postoperatively, and the hinged knee brace is discontinued at 12 weeks postoperatively.

We have experienced only one postoperative patellar tendon rupture in more than 1,300 ACL reconstructions. Based on this experience, we continue to advocate use of a drop-lock hinged knee brace for the first 6 weeks postoperatively to protect the donor site.

Management of Patellar Tendinitis

Patellar tendinitis is a distinct cause of postoperative anterior knee pain following ACL reconstruction and is not necessarily related to postoperative knee stiffness. It is commonly seen at approximately 3 months after the index procedure in patients progressing quickly with rehabilitation. We believe that clinical progress and an increasing activity level in these patients outpace the recovery of quadriceps strength and will result in patellar tendinitis. This problem invariably resolves as thigh strength increases, and patellar tendinitis is unusual more than 1 year postoperatively. Symptoms can be minimized with a Chopat strap and an added rehabilitation focus on hamstrings flexibility and eccentric quadriceps exercises. Local anti-inflammatory medications may also speed recovery. We are not aware of any literature that specifically attributes postoperative patellar tendinitis to autologous patellar tendon harvest, although we see this problem clinically in this subgroup of patients. Furthermore, no literature relates postoperative tendinitis among patients who have had central-third patellar tendon harvests to closure of the residual tendon defect rather than leaving the defect open.

MANAGEMENT AND OUTCOME SUMMARY

At the time of surgery, the fracture was confirmed at the proximal aspect of the harvest bed, and an anatomic reduction was obtained. Postoperatively, the patient was braced in full extension. Physical therapy was initiated with a focus on prone heel hangs, extension board use, and immediate non–weight-bearing flexion. Weight bearing with the brace locked in extension was allowed. At 8 weeks postoperatively, radiographs revealed fracture healing and maintenance of an anatomic reduction. The brace was discontinued, and closed chain quadriceps exercises were initiated. After continued physical therapy, the patient recovered symmetric range of motion, and hardware removal was scheduled.

STRATEGIES TO MINIMIZE COMPLICATIONS

Macrotraumatic extensor mechanism disruptions are uncommon following ACL reconstruction; however, they are significant complications that often require reoperation. Intraoperative precision when harvesting the patellar tendon and implementation of contemporary postoperative rehabilitation and bracing protocols can minimize their occurrence.

REFERENCES

1. Ferrari JD, Bush-Joseph CA, Bach BR Jr: Endoscopic anterior cruciate ligament reconstruction with patellar tendon autograft: Surgical technique. *Tech Orthop* 1998;13:262-274.
2. Miyasaka KC, Daniel DM, Stone ML, et al: The incidence of knee ligament injuries in the general population. *Am J Knee Surg* 1991;5:3-8.
3. Freedman KB, D'Amato M, Nedeff D, et al: Comparison of patellar tendon and hamstring ACL reconstruction: A metaanalysis. *Am J Sports Med* 2003;31:2-11.
4. Buss DD, Min R, Skyhar M, et al: Nonoperative treatment of anterior cruciate ligament injuries in a selected group of patients. *Am J Sports Med* 1995;23:160-165.
5. Shelbourne KD, Trumper RV: Preventing anterior knee pain after anterior cruciate ligament reconstruction. *Am J Sports Med* 1997;25:41-47.
6. Brownstein B, Bronner S: Patella fractures associated with accelerated ACL rehabilitation in patients with autogenous patella tendon reconstructions. *J Orthop Sports Phys Ther* 1997;26:168-172.
7. Christen B, Jakob RP: Fractures associated with patellar ligament grafts in cruciate ligament surgery. *J Bone Joint Surg Br* 1992;74:617-620.
8. Viola R, Vianello R: Three cases of patella fracture in 1,320 anterior cruciate ligament reconstructions with bone-patellar tendon-bone autograft. *Arthroscopy* 1999;15:93-97.
9. Berg EE: Management of patella fractures associated with central third bone-patella tendon-bone autograft ACL reconstructions. *Arthroscopy* 1996;12:756-759.
10. Moholkar K, Taylor D, O'Reagan M, et al: A biomechanical analysis of four different methods of harvesting bone-patellar tendon-bone graft in porcine knees. *J Bone Joint Surg Am* 2002;84:1782-1787.
11. Shapiro JD, Cohn BT, Jackson DW, et al: The biomechanical effects of geometric configuration of bone-tendon-bone autografts in anterior cruciate ligament reconstruction. *Arthroscopy* 1992;8:453-458.
12. DuMontier TA, Metcalf MH, Simonian PT, et al: Patella fracture after anterior cruciate ligament reconstruction with the patellar tendon: A comparison between different shaped bone block excisions. *Am J Knee Surg* 2001;14:9-15.
13. Daluga D, Johnson C, Bach BR Jr: Primary bone grafting following graft procurement for anterior

cruciate ligament insufficiency. *Arthroscopy* 1990;6:205-208.

14. Tsuda E, Okamura Y, Ishibashi Y, et al: Techniques for reducing anterior knee symptoms after anterior cruciate ligament reconstruction using a bone-patellar tendon-bone autograft. *Am J Sports Med* 2001;29:450-456.

15. Marumoto JM, Mitsunaga MM, Richardson AB, et al: Late patellar tendon ruptures after removal of the central third for anterior cruciate ligament reconstruction. *Am J Sports Med* 1996;24:698-702.

16. McMaster PE: Tendon and muscle ruptures: Clinical and experimental studies on the causes and location of subcutaneous ruptures. *J Bone Joint Surg Am* 1933;15: 705-722.

Chapter 4

Septic Arthritis Following ACL Reconstruction

Jeffrey J. Kovacic, MD
Richard D. Parker, MD
Kurt P. Spindler, MD

Case Presentation

History

A 28-year-old man who sustained a noncontact twisting injury to his right knee while playing softball reported feeling and hearing a pop during the injury; he subsequently noted that his knee locked, and he initially had a difficult time with ambulation. He also reported knee swelling over the next 24 hours. He was evaluated initially in a local emergency department where he was treated with ice, a knee immobilizer, and crutches. He presented for specialty evaluation the following week.

The patient had no significant past medical or surgical history. He was not taking any medications, he denied any previous injury to the affected knee, and his occupation required only sedentary activities at a desk. His recreational activities included softball and triathlon.

During the physical examination, the patient's left knee was noted to be in neutral alignment, asymptomatic, and stable to stress in all planes and with rotation. Range of motion in this knee was 0°, 0°, and 140°. The affected right knee had a 2+ effusion with a range of motion of 0°, 10°, and 120°. He also had isolated medial joint line tenderness and a positive Lachman test. The pivot-shift test could not be performed because of profound medial joint line pain; however, valgus laxity at 0° and 30° was equal to that of the contralateral knee. The right knee had no varus laxity or increased external rotation. The posterior cruciate ligament was found to be intact by examination with a hard end point.

Radiographs of the patient's knees were negative. MRI revealed a large, displaced, peripheral bucket-handle medial meniscal tear resting in the intercondylar notch and complete disruption of the anterior cruciate ligament (ACL). Femoral and tibial bone bruising without obvious articular cartilage disruption also was noted.

Treatment options were discussed with the patient, and he chose simultaneous surgical repair of the medial meniscus and ACL reconstruction. Surgery was performed 19 days after the date of injury. Examination under anesthesia confirmed the physical examination findings, and diagnostic arthroscopy revealed a complete tear of the ACL and a tear of the medial meniscus at the meniscocapsular junction. The lateral meniscus and the articular cartilage were intact.

Surgery consisted of endoscopic reconstruction of the ACL with autologous bone-patellar tendon-bone (BTB) graft through standard anteromedial and anterolateral portals. Femoral fixation was performed using an EndoButton (Smith & Nephew Endoscopy, Andover, MA), and the tibial side was fixed with a cannulated interference screw. The medial meniscus was reduced and repaired using an inside-out technique with nonabsorbable No. 2-0 suture. A drain was placed intra-articularly before completion of the procedure, and the patient was given 1 g of cefazolin preoperatively and 1 g postoperatively. A tourniquet was applied but not inflated during the procedure. The procedure was performed without difficulty or complication.

Current Problem and Treatment

When the patient was seen on postoperative day 3 he had no evidence of infection or deep vein thrombosis. However, when he presented for routine follow-up 1 week later, the patient had a temperature of 101.5° (39°C), flu-like symptoms, and severe pain in the treated knee. Additional findings at this time included knee effusion and warmth and painful range of motion of 0°, 10°, and 80° in the affected knee and 0°, 0°, and 130° in the normal opposite knee. The treated knee was aspirated, and 10 mL of blood-tinged synovial fluid was sent for Gram stain, culture, and sensitivity. Analysis of the synovial fluid showed a white blood cell (WBC) count of 55,000 mm^3 (85% polymorphonuclear cells), no crystals, and few gram-positive cocci. Infection with methicillin-sensitive *Staphylococcus aureus* was later identified. The patient was taken emergently to the operating room for irrigation and débridement of the septic knee.

Surgery began with an evaluation under anesthesia. Range of motion was 0°, 0°, and 80°. Next, all surgical wounds were opened, irrigated with 10 L of normal saline solution under pulse lavage, and then débrided. Subsequently, an arthroscopic synovectomy was performed, and the joint was irrigated with 24 L of normal saline solution. No purulence was noted on arthroscopy. Several cultures were obtained and sent for microbiologic analysis. The ACL graft did not appear infected (**Figure 1**). The tibial screw was removed and sterilized, and the tibial tunnel was irrigated. The graft was tensioned by hand and the screw

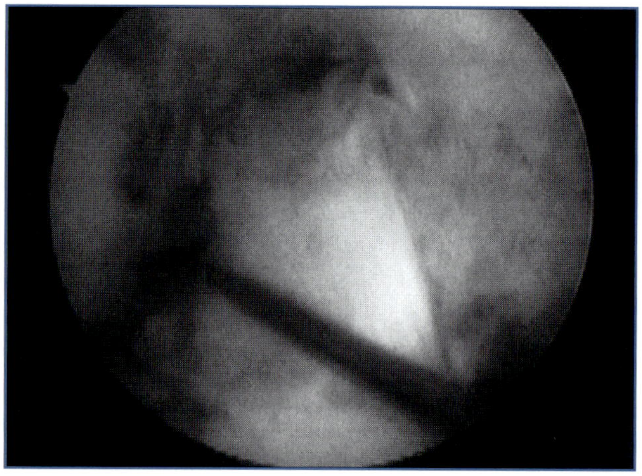

Figure 1 Arthroscopic images at the initial irrigation and débridement showing an intact BTB ACL graft, as indicated by the probe.

replaced. Range of motion at the end of the procedure was 0°, 0°, and 140°. The wounds were loosely closed over packing, and an intra-articular drain was placed. The patient was admitted to the hospital, intravenous (IV) antibiotics were started, and an infectious disease consultation was initiated.

Discussion

Recognizing the Problem

Septic arthritis after ACL reconstruction is uncommon, with a reported rate between 0.14% and 1.7%.[1-7] In a systematic review of nine randomized controlled trials of autograft choice (level of evidence, 1), the overall infection rate was 0.8% (n = 5/608).[8] However, outcomes were not analyzed separately for these patients. Thus, the possibility of a 1% incidence of septic arthritis after autograft ACL reconstructions with patellar tendon or hamstrings grafts should be discussed preoperatively with all patients. Higher infection rates have been reported with the use of synthetic graft materials, but these have since fallen out of favor. Other factors that appear to increase the risk of septic arthritis after ACL reconstruction include a history of previous surgery to the affected knee and performing concomitant procedures (ie, meniscal repair).[2,3] Graft type (hamstrings versus BTB), tourniquet use, and a one- versus two-incision technique do not appear to influence the incidence of septic arthritis.[3] Many surgeons favor preoperative prophylaxis with antibiotics, based on the work of Schurman and associates,[9] who reported that preoperative antibiotics protected the rabbit joint from a low-dose bacterial challenge.

Septic arthritis following ACL reconstruction typically presents with a sudden increase in pain, elevated temperature (greater than 100°F [38°C]), and knee effusion, warmth, and painful limited range of motion. Occasionally, there may be drainage from surgical wounds. However, if the pyarthrosis is caused by a less virulent organism such as coagulase-negative *Staphylococcus*, the clinical presentation may appear more indolent.[7] These infections commonly present less obviously than a native septic arthritis. If a change in postoperative course is noted, such as significantly reduced motion in physical therapy or increased postoperative pain, septic arthritis should be suspected, and the knee should be aspirated. Although the time from the index procedure to the onset of symptoms can vary from days to months, most infections that are reported present within 20 days of the reconstruction.

If septic arthritis is suspected clinically, immediate joint aspiration and laboratory studies are indicated. Synovial fluid is often turbid and yellow, and the synovial fluid WBC count can range from less than 10,000 to 150,000/mm^3 but usually is more than 50,000/mm^3 with more than 90% polymorphonuclear cells. Fluid cultures often reveal the offending organism, typically *S aureus* or *S epidermidis*, but other bacteria and fungi have been reported.[10] Antibiotic sensitivities are useful for guiding antimicrobial therapy. The length of IV or subsequent antibiotic treatment has not been clearly defined; therefore, we recommend consulting an infectious disease specialist for guidance. We would rather overtreat an infection than risk recurrence, provided that few side effects are associated with the antibiotic selected. Erythrocyte sedimentation rate and C-reactive protein have the highest negative predictive value for septic arthritis; however, these values often remain elevated during the first week after uncomplicated ACL reconstruction.[7,11] Although the absolute peripheral WBC count is notoriously unreliable in this setting, a left shift commonly is observed in the differential WBC count.

Management of Septic Arthritis

Once the diagnosis is confirmed, prompt irrigation and débridement of affected tissue is indicated. Although open arthrotomy is an option, arthroscopic irrigation and débridement has become widely accepted as an effective method for treating pyarthrosis with less morbidity.1 We have successfully treated infections with an arthroscopic-only approach. In addition to partial or total synovectomy, all associated surgical wounds should be opened and treated with irrigation and débridement to prevent infection and the potential for an extra-articular abscess, which could lead to reinoculation of the joint. These wounds should be left open or closed loosely over packing or drains. Any foreign material (ie, sutures, hardware) that is no longer required to secure fixation should be removed, especially if the graft has incorporated into bone tunnels.

During arthroscopy, special attention must be paid to the ACL graft. The decision to remove the ACL graft currently is being debated, and published data (level of evidence, 5) are insufficient to guide treatment decisions. Authors who favor graft removal argue that until the graft incorporates and revascularizes, it acts as a nonviable foreign body that is capable of harboring bacteria, sterile microbial fragments, and inflammatory mediators that could contribute to chondrolysis.[2,4] Burks and associates[4] reported excellent results with this approach but acknowledge it requires another surgery to revise the ACL reconstruction.

Reports of graft retention are mixed. Even though infections can be eradicated successfully with the graft in place, some authors report inferior outcomes compared with uncomplicated ACL reconstruction.[3,7] However, these outcomes were likely secondary to articular cartilage damage as a result of infection and/or additional surgical procedures rather than a result of graft incompetence. In contrast, Viola and associates[1] reported outcomes similar to those of uncomplicated ACL reconstruction. Their 13 patients were managed initially with only joint aspiration and antibiotics. Irrigation and débridement was performed only if patients did not respond to initial treatment. Long-term follow-up has not been reported.

Based on case series in the literature and our experience, we recommend the following approach to management of septic arthritis after ACL reconstruction. At the first signs and symptoms of infection, immediate joint aspiration and laboratory analysis are indicated, specifically C-reactive protein, erythrocyte sedimentation rate, and WBC count with differential. Empiric antibiotics should be administered until the culture results are known. With strong suspicion or confirmation of the diagnosis, arthroscopic irrigation and débridement with synovectomy should be performed. All associated wounds should be opened, débrided, and any foreign material removed.

Graft retention can be considered if the diagnosis has not been delayed, the joint appears benign, and the graft appears viable and without gross infection. If the infection appears established or if there has been a delay in diagnosis, graft and hardware removal should be strongly considered. The joint and associated wounds should be drained postoperatively, IV antibiotics should be continued, and an infectious disease consultation obtained. If graft retention is elected, repeat irrigation and débridement is warranted if a poor response to treatment ensues, and the graft should be removed because the integrity of the articular cartilage is the priority.

Four to 6 weeks of antibiotics typically follow, with the route of administration dependent on the organism and the antibiotic chosen. Antibiotic treatment should be individualized based on patient response and the recommendation of the infectious disease specialist.

Postoperative rehabilitation should consist of an initial period of non–weight-bearing status while maintaining range of motion. Continuous passive motion devices need not be used unless arthrofibrosis develops. After the infection resolves, development of an arthrofibrotic reaction that requires aggressive management is not uncommon.

If graft removal is necessary, Burks and associates[4] report excellent results with early reimplantation of an ACL graft. They successfully revised their reconstructions within 6 weeks of eradicating infection. They harvested autologous, ipsilateral BTB or hamstrings grafts in each of their four patients. Their preferred preoperative prophylaxis was the antibiotic used to eradicate the previous infection.

Management and Outcome Summary

The patient in the case study required two arthroscopic irrigation and débridement procedures to eradicate the infection. He was maintained on 2 g of IV cefazolin every 8 hours for 42 days at the recommendation of the infectious disease consultant. This was followed by another 28 days of oral cephalexin, 500 mg four times a day.

His postoperative course was complicated by arthrofibrosis, which limited his range of motion to 0°, 0°, and 60° despite aggressive physical therapy (four times per week). He underwent arthroscopic adhesiolysis with manipulation 7 months after the last irrigation and débridement. At the same time, the tibial interference screw, EndoButton, and sutures were removed. The ACL graft was found to be intact and competent, and the bone plugs were well incorporated. Cultures obtained during the procedure were negative. Full range of motion was obtained at the conclusion of the procedure. Postoperatively, he was admitted for epidural analgesia and physical therapy, which included the use of continuous passive motion.

Over the next several years, the patient was closely followed clinically and radiographically. He has not had any sign of recurrent infection or osteomyelitis, knee range of motion was 0°, 0°, and 135°, and his knee has remained stable in all planes. However, he reported considerable pain with weight bearing, localized to the medial compartment of the affected knee for about 2 years. Radiographs at the time revealed well-maintained joint spaces but mild osteophyte formation in all three compartments and irregularity in the medial femoral condyle and tibial plateau on the 45° flexion weight-bearing view. MRI at the time revealed changes in the medial femoral condyle consistent with osteonecrosis (**Figure 2**). The repaired medial meniscus and ACL graft were intact. Management at this time consisted of observation and a valgus-producing unloading brace. His pain eventually resolved.

Approximately 5 years after ACL reconstruction, the patient's right knee was asymptomatic and functioning normally. Radiographs revealed mild progression of the joint space narrowing and osteophyte formation in all three compartments. MRI revealed irregularities in the articular cartilage.

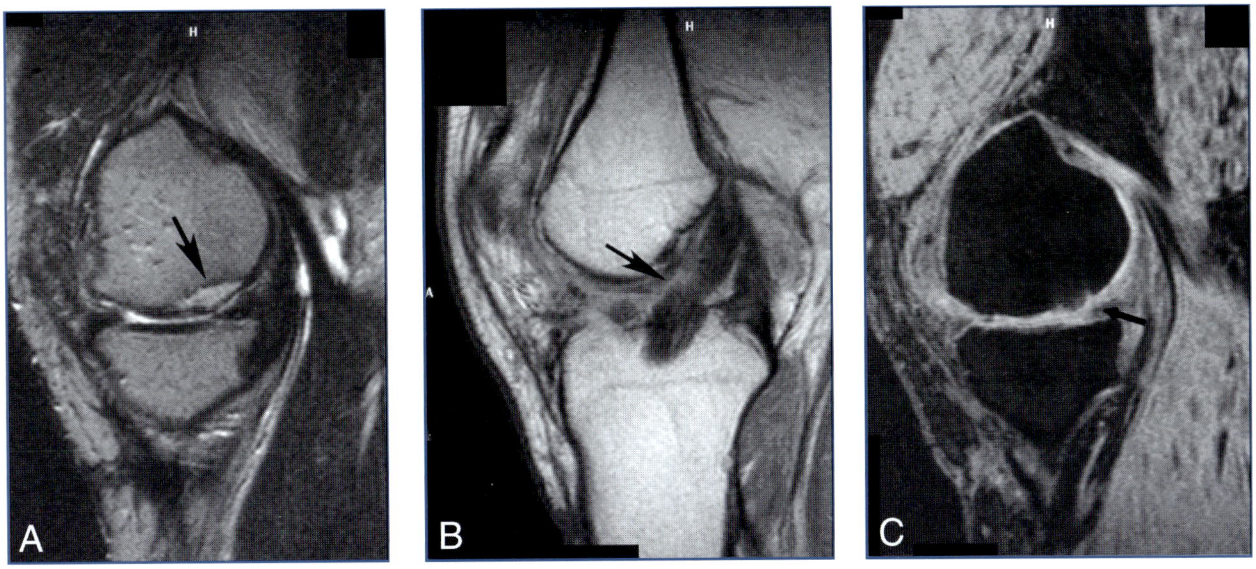

Figure 2 MRI scans show the zone of osteonecrosis **(A,** arrow**)**, an intact ACL graft **(B,** arrow**)**, and an articular cartilage irregularity consistent with chondrolysis **(C,** arrow**)**.

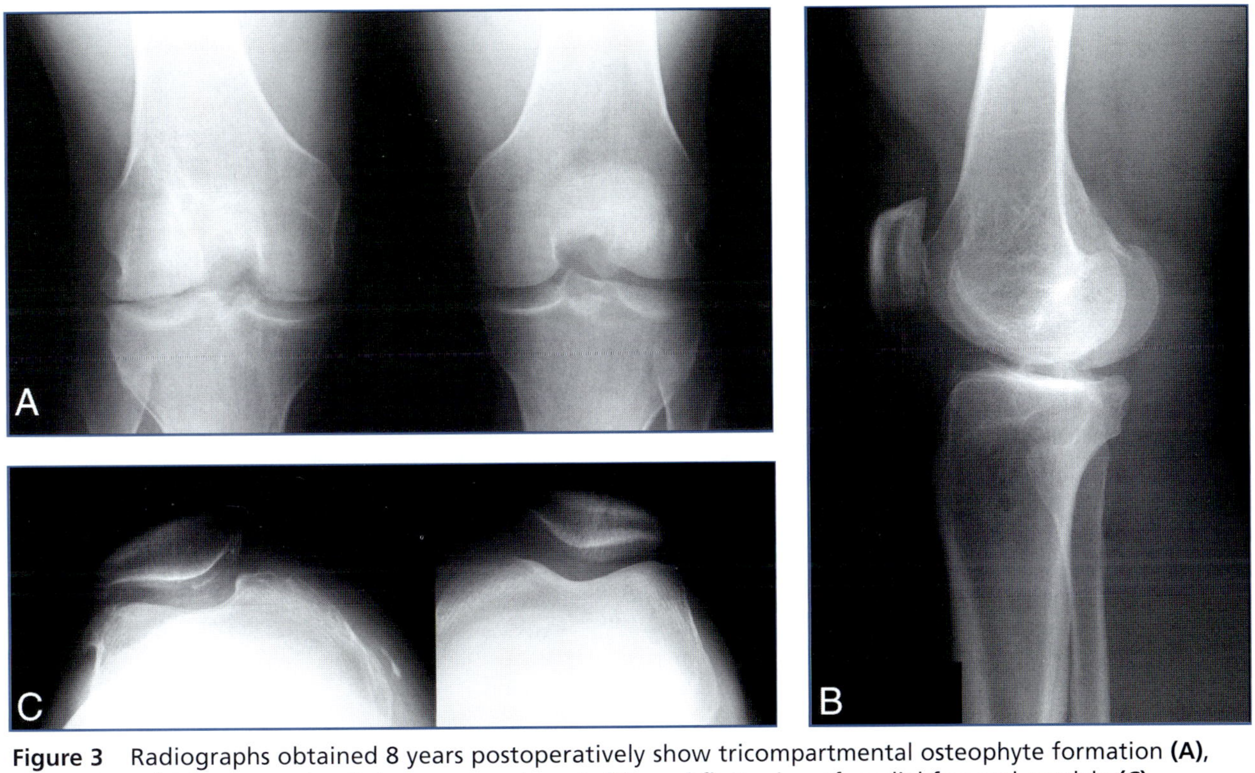

Figure 3 Radiographs obtained 8 years postoperatively show tricompartmental osteophyte formation **(A)**, narrowing of joint spaces in all three compartments **(B)**, and flattening of medial femoral condyle **(C)**.

However, the ACL and menisci were intact, and there was no evidence of ongoing osteonecrosis.

Eight years after ACL reconstruction, the patient was involved in triathlon activities. His most recent radiographs are shown in **Figure 3**. The degenerative changes in his knee are slowly progressing, but he is functioning at a high level.

Strategies to Prevent Common Complications

Overall, the goals of eradicating the septic arthritis and restoring function with a stable knee were achieved. However, we believe the integrity of the patient's articular cartilage was compromised as a result of the infectious process that developed after the initial ACL reconstruction, despite early recognition and aggressive treatment. This case illustrates several potential sequelae of postoperative septic arthritis, including arthrofibrosis, osteonecrosis, and articular cartilage degeneration. In this situation, priority should be given to eradication of the infection, then to articular cartilage preservation, then to maintenance of range of motion, and last to the graft. By adhering to this approach, the best possible outcome can be achieved.

References

1. Viola R, Marzano N, Vianello R: An unusual epidemic of Staphylococcus-negative infections involving anterior cruciate ligament reconstruction with salvage of the graft and function. *Arthroscopy* 2000;16:173-177.
2. Williams RJ III, Laurencin CT, Warren RF, Speciale AC, Brause BD, O'Brien S: Septic arthritis after arthroscopic anterior cruciate ligament reconstruction: Diagnosis and management. *Am J Sports Med* 1997;25:261-267.
3. McAllister DR, Parker RD, Cooper AE, Recht MP, Abate J: Outcomes of postoperative septic arthritis after anterior cruciate ligament reconstruction. *Am J Sports Med* 1999;27:562-570.
4. Burks RT, Friederichs MG, Fink B, Luker MG, West HS, Greis PE: Treatment of postoperative anterior cruciate ligament infections with graft removal and early reimplantation. *Am J Sports Med* 2003;31:414-418.
5. Indelli PF, Dillingham M, Fanton G, Schurman DJ: Septic arthritis in postoperative anterior cruciate ligament reconstruction. *Clin Orthop* 2002;398:182-188.
6. Fong SY, Tan JL: Septic arthritis after arthroscopic anterior cruciate ligament reconstruction. *Ann Acad Med Singapore* 2004;33:228-234.
7. Schollin-Borg M, Michaelsson K, Rahme H: Presentation, outcome, and cause of septic arthritis after anterior cruciate ligament reconstruction: A case control study. *Arthroscopy* 2003;19:941-947.
8. Spindler KP, Kuhn JE, Freedman KB, Matthews CE, Dittus RS, Harrell FE Jr: ACL reconstruction autograft choice: Bone-tendon-bone vs hamstring. Does it really matter? A systematic review. *Am J Sports Med* 2004;32:1986-1995.
9. Schurman DJ, Johnson BL Jr, Amstutz HC: Knee joint infections with Staphylococcus aureus and Micrococcus species. *J Bone Joint Surg Am* 1975;57:40-49.
10. Burke WV, Zych GA: Fungal infection following replacement of the anterior cruciate ligament: A case report. *J Bone Joint Surg Am* 2002;84:449-453.
11. Margheritini F, Camillieri G, Mancini L, Mariana PP: C-reactive protein and erythrocyte sedimentation rate changes following arthroscopically assisted anterior cruciate ligament reconstruction. *Knee Surg Sports Traumatol Arthrosc* 2001;9:343-345.

Chapter 5

Arthrofibrosis Following ACL Reconstruction

Pietro Tonino, MD
Randall J. Risinger, MD
Michael Garcia, MD
Bernard R. Bach, Jr, MD

Case Presentation

History

A 43-year-old tennis player who sustained a twisting hyperflexion injury to his left knee felt an immediate pop and effusion. At initial presentation, the patient held his knee flexed 15° and was unable to extend it further, the extensor mechanism was intact, the patellar examination was unremarkable, and knee flexion was 100° secondary to a 1+ effusion. He had a grade IIB Lachman test and guarding with attempts at pivot-shift testing. KT-1000 arthrometric (MEDmetric Corp, San Diego, CA) testing revealed an 8-mm side-to-side maximum manual difference.

The knee radiographs were normal. MRI revealed an effusion, an anterior cruciate ligament (ACL) disruption with classic lateral compartment bone bruises, and a bucket-handle medial meniscus tear displaced into the intercondylar notch.

The patient was counseled about both nonsurgical and surgical treatment options. Based on his desire to continue sports participation for more than 6 hours a week in activities that would put his knee at risk for further pivoting episodes and a high (> 6 mm) KT-1000 arthrometric side-to-side difference, ACL reconstruction was recommended. Initial meniscal surgery to facilitate motion recovery and staged ACL reconstruction also were discussed.

By 12 days after the injury, the patient had achieved significant gains in range of motion (ROM), lacking only 2° of terminal extension and flexion beyond 125°; therefore, a single-stage procedure was selected. After a complete discussion with the patient about graft alternatives, a patellar tendon autograft was chosen.

The patient underwent an uncomplicated arthroscopically assisted ACL reconstruction and medial meniscus repair 21 days after the injury. A standard single-incision endoscopic reconstruction technique[1] was used, and an inside-out meniscus repair was performed using an accessory incision. Diagnostic arthroscopy did not reveal any other significant intra-articular pathology.

The patient was discharged home from the recovery room after physical therapy instruction, and the initial postoperative recovery was uneventful. The postoperative rehabilitation goals during the first 6 weeks were (1) unassisted full weight bearing by 10 days with the knee braced and (2) full knee extension by 1 week and 120° of flexion by 6 weeks postoperatively. These goals typically are met with home exercises for the first 7 to 10 days followed by formal supervised physical therapy.

Current Problem and Treatment

Radiographs obtained at the time of suture removal revealed appropriate tunnel and interference screw positions. The patient had complete hyperextension and flexion to 90°. However, at the 6-week postoperative follow-up, he lacked 10° of full extension, and flexion measured 110°. Therefore, a methylprednisolone dose pack and nonsteroidal anti-inflammatory medication (NSAIDs) were prescribed, and use of a knee extension board was stressed during subsequent physical therapy sessions. By 12 weeks postoperatively, ROM had improved to 8° to 130°. However, despite continued aggressive physical therapy, subsequent follow-up revealed no improvement in the 8° flexion contracture; the normal, unaffected right knee hyperextended 2°. The patient regained full flexion equal to the contralateral knee; however, he reported that he could not lock out his quadriceps and noticed anterior knee pain with increasing physical activity.

Because of persistent symptomatic loss of terminal extension, the patient underwent examination under anesthesia and arthroscopic débridement 9 months after the index procedure. Examination at this time revealed a persistent 8° flexion contracture and diminished patellar mobility. On subsequent arthroscopic evaluation, a superolateral viewing portal had to be created initially because significant scar tissue was encountered during attempts to create an inferolateral portal. Arthroscopic findings included bands of scar tissue in the suprapatellar pouch, scar tissue extending directly from the patellar articular margin into both the medial and lateral gutters, fat pad scarring with evidence of partial adherence to the medial femoral condyle, and a cyclops nodule (**Figure 1**).

Discussion

Recognizing the Problem and Situations at Risk

Recognizing Arthrofibrosis

If not recognized early and treated aggressively, postoperative loss of motion and associated anterior knee pain can be more disabling than the initial symptoms that led to the ACL reconstruction. The overall prevalence of abnormal motion after ACL reconstruction reportedly has ranged from 4% in contemporary studies to 35% historically.[2] Intraoperative precision and perioperative care have evolved as understanding of the risk factors associated with motion loss has improved, minimizing this complication.

Although normal knee ROM varies among individuals, most people have some degree of hyperextension, with an average of 5° of recurvatum in men and 6° in women.[3] Hyperextension of the knee is necessary because it permits the normal kinematics of the screw-home mechanism and relaxation of the quadriceps muscle during the stance phase. Most patients find loss of extension more problematic than loss of flexion; relatively small extension deficits necessitate increased quadriceps activity, place increased strain on the patellofemoral joint, and produce anterior knee pain. As little as a 5° loss of terminal extension has been associated with patellofemoral pain and a limp; unfortunately, this degree of extension loss has been reported in 5% to 13% of patients after ACL reconstruction.[4] A 10° loss of terminal extension diminishes running speed, which is not well tolerated by active individuals, and a 20° loss may cause a functional limb-length discrepancy. In contrast, restricted flexion does not affect gait as long as the knee can be flexed at least 60°.[4] Thus, regaining postoperative hyperextension equal to the contralateral knee is critical.

Historically, any patient presenting with loss of motion after knee trauma or reconstructive surgery has been diagnosed as having arthrofibrosis. However, throughout the literature, this umbrella diagnosis has been given to many different discrete pathologies; thus, there is no universally accepted definition of this condition, and the true incidence of arthrofibrosis following ACL reconstruction is difficult to ascertain.

Defining Arthrofibrosis Arthrofibrosis can be categorized into three main types of lesions that vary in severity, presentation, and incidence. First, the cyclops lesion, or local arthrofibrosis, is described as a localized nodule of intra-articular arthrofibrosis located anterolateral to the tibial tunnel of the reconstructed ACL. It attaches to the graft and the tibia, resulting in a mechanical block to extension only[5]

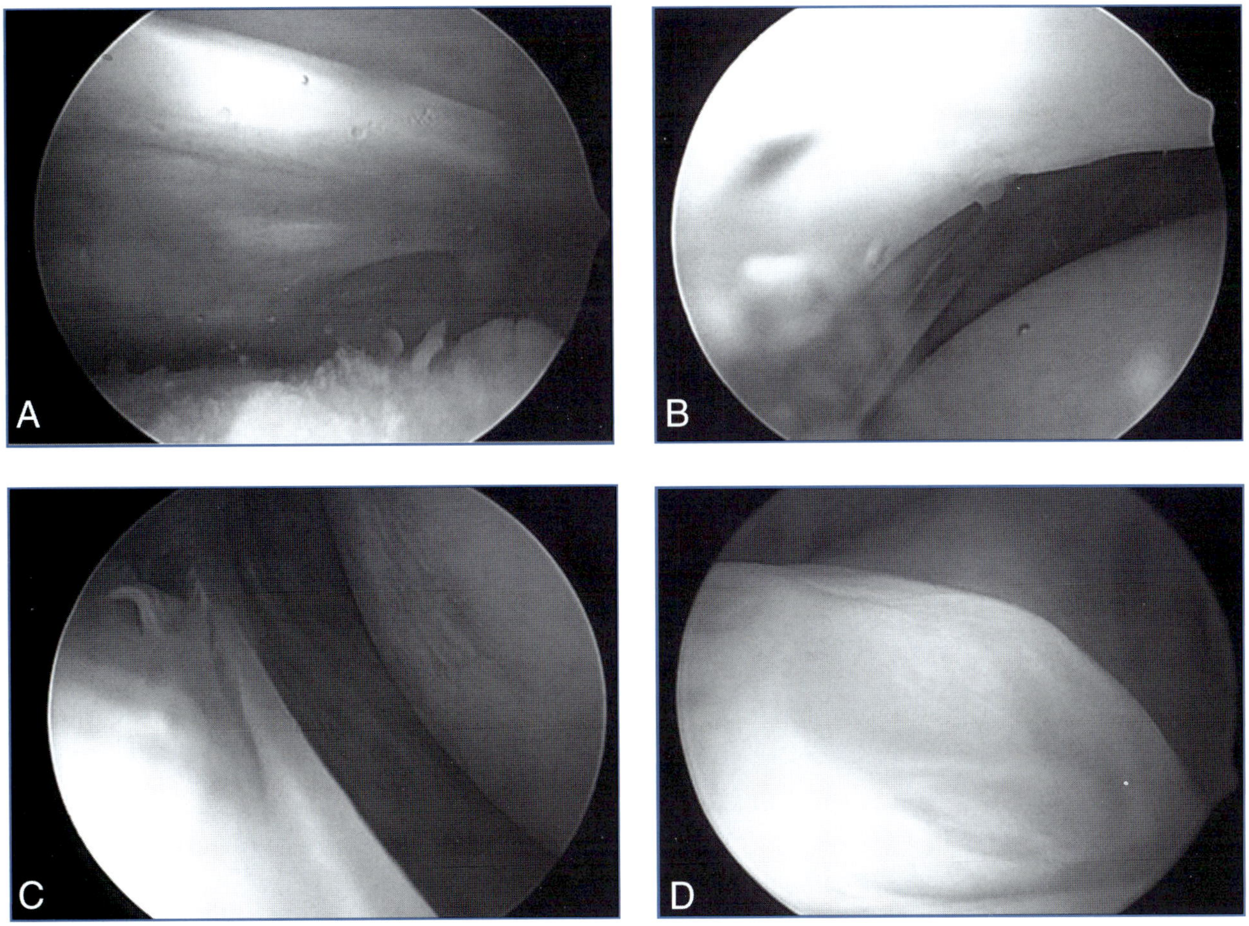

Figure 1 Arthroscopic images showing a fibrous band in the suprapatellar pouch **(A)**, a scar extending from the lateral nonarticular patellar margin into the lateral gutter **(B)**, an anteromedial scar with evidence of adherence to the medial femoral condyle **(C)**, and a cyclops lesion **(D)**.

and is the most commonly described cause of loss of extension.

In infrapatellar contracture syndrome, the fat pad becomes fibrotic with inferior translation of the patella, limited patellar mobility, and loss of knee flexion and extension.[6] Global arthrofibrosis, the least common type, is characterized by loss of flexion and extension with fibrosis of the medial and lateral gutters and the suprapatellar pouch.[6] Extracapsular fibrosis may be evident as well and is associated with the worst prognosis.

Classifying Arthrofibrosis Shelbourne and associates[7] described a classification system for arthrofibrosis based on the pattern and severity of knee stiffness. Patients with type I have normal flexion and less than 10° extension loss; patients with type II have normal flexion and more than 10° extension loss. Patients with type III have a combined flexion loss of more than 25° and an extension loss of more than 10° with decreased patellar mobility, and patients with type IV have an extension loss of more than 10°, total flexion of less than 120°, and infrapatellar contracture syndrome.[7]

Patella infera or baja can be seen postoperatively and is caused by both extrinsic and intrinsic mechanisms. Whether closure of the defect following central-third patellar tendon harvest contributes to

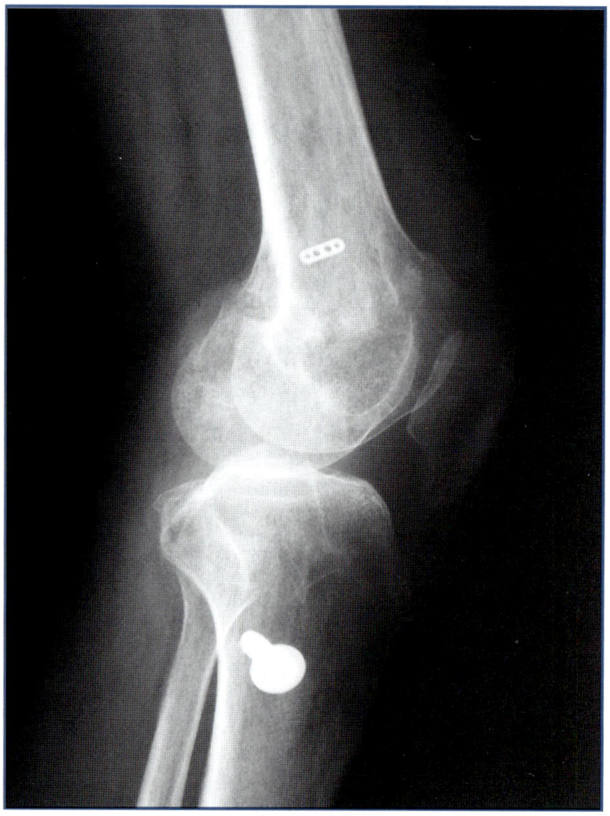

Figure 2 Lateral radiograph showing infrapatellar contracture syndrome. Note the evidence of a healed supracondylar femur fracture sustained during a prior knee manipulation. (Courtesy of Charles A. Bush-Joseph, MD.)

this condition remains debatable. Localized fibroproliferation and scarring of peripatellar and fat pad tissues, which can occur in the presence of patella baja, combined with quadriceps muscle weakness, can exacerbate patellar entrapment and result in significantly restricted extension and flexion. Paulos and associates[8] were among the first to describe this variation of arthrofibrosis and termed it infrapatellar contracture syndrome (**Figure 2**). The anterior fat pad becomes densely scarred and adherent to the underlying tibia, significantly altering both patellofemoral and tibiofemoral contact and kinematics.[9] Quadriceps inhibition causes additional distal patellar migration, and intrinsic tendon shortening can be pronounced. This combination of abnormalities invariably produces anterior knee pain, and, with time, patellofemoral arthritis can develop.[10]

Scarring of the posterior capsule and contracture of the posterior soft tissues results in a true knee flexion contracture. The contracture usually is secondary to prolonged immobilization or prolonged loss of extension from another cause that has been left untreated. However, flexion contractures can occur following meniscal repair if sutures are not secured with the knee in full extension. Tying sutures with the knee flexed will plicate the posterior capsule and effectively capture the knee, resulting in diminished posterior capsular volume.

Primary Blocks to Terminal Extension A localized fibroproliferative process anterior to the tibial tunnel is the most common pathology unique to ACL reconstructions that causes loss of motion. Jackson and Schaefer[11] were the first to describe this scar nodule, or cyclops lesion, which was noted to develop in 2% to 4% of ACL reconstructions. Histologically, this process is dominated by fibroblasts and an abundant scar response; cellular metaplasia can occur over time with chondrocyte development and fibrocartilage production within the lesion. The early fibrous hyperplasia seen in cyclops lesions resembles arthrofibrosis histologically, but these lesions clearly represent a distinct pathologic process.

Cyclops lesions typically are attached to the graft and soft tissue overlying the anterior tibia (**Figure 3**). With extension, impingement of this nodule occurs in the intercondylar notch, causing a painless clunk and blocking terminal extension. Two etiologies for these nodules have been proposed: (1) primary graft impingement from an anteriorized tibial tunnel or inadequate notchplasty results in graft injury and subsequent nodule formation;[12] or (2) debris in the form of bone from reaming of the tibial tunnel or residual native ACL stump left at the time of index procedure causes a natural fibroproliferative response and subsequent nodule formation.[13] Some researchers believe that achieving terminal hyperextension in the early postoperative period may prevent nodule formation, regardless of the etiology, because the ACL graft will be well seated in the intercondylar notch and will not provide space for nodule growth.[14]

Central bony proliferations also are common blocks to terminal extension. Anterior tibial inter-

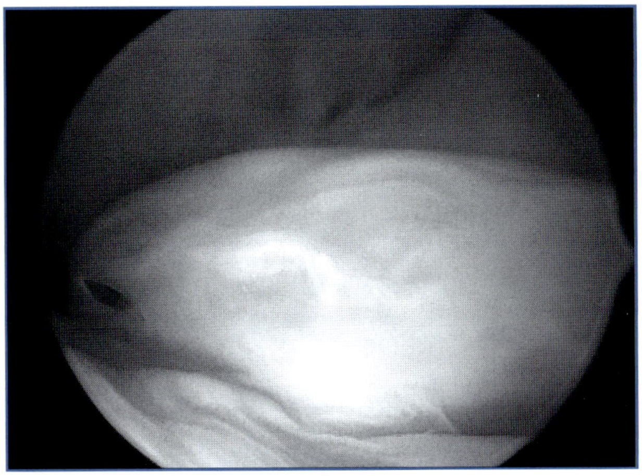

Figure 3 Arthroscopic image showing a cyclops lesion in the left knee as seen from the inferolateral viewing portal. The intact graft is seen in the background.

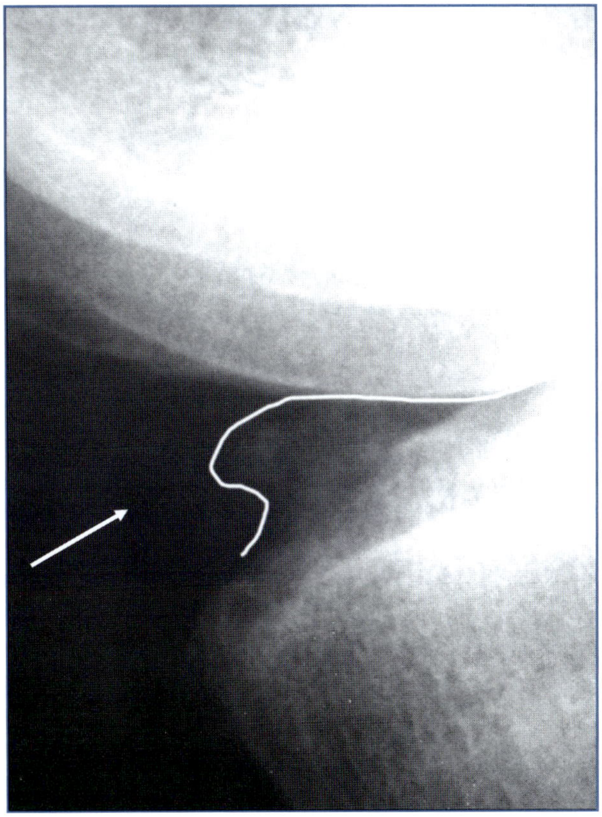

Figure 4
Lateral radiograph showing an anterior tibial intercondylar eminence ("anvil") osteophyte (arrow), which limits terminal extension.

condylar eminence osteophytes are the most frequent finding and, when present, are visualized clearly on radiographs (**Figure 4**). Notch regrowth or hypertrophy also can occur despite adequate index notchplasty and similar block extension.

Risk Factors for Arthrofibrosis

In a patient undergoing ACL reconstruction, several factors in the perioperative period have been associated with ultimate loss of knee motion and poor clinical outcomes: (1) poor preoperative ROM and inflammation combined with early surgery; (2) graft malposition or lack of isometry; (3) excessive graft tension, especially if nonisometric; (4) inadequate notchplasty; (5) associated meniscal repair with potential capture of the joint capsule; (6) concomitant extra-articular injury or procedures; (7) poor postoperative rehabilitation or excessive immobilization; (8) complex regional pain syndrome (CRPS); (9) neurapraxia related to the use of a tourniquet; and (10) infection. At least half of these risk factors can be modified and effectively eliminated.

Timing of Surgery Shelbourne and associates[7,15,16] evaluated the correlation between early ACL reconstruction and arthrofibrosis. In a retrospective study of 169 patients, the authors reported a significant increase in the incidence of loss of extension in patients who underwent surgery within 3 weeks of their injury. Cosgarea and associates[17] also reported a significantly higher risk for arthrofibrosis in patients undergoing ACL reconstruction within 3 weeks of their injury.

Extra-articular swelling, warmth, size of effusion, severity of pain, and ROM can be monitored to assess the degree of inflammation about the joint, with ROM the easiest parameter to assess.[6] This monitoring can help determine the optimal time for surgery. Some authors believe that the resolution of soft-tissue inflammation and effusion and early motion recovery are indicators for acceptable early surgical reconstruction.[18]

Injury Mechanism Shapiro and Freedman[19] reported higher rates of motion loss associated with multiple ligament injuries. Motion problems were noted in 30% of patients with traumatic knee dislocations and in 57% of patients who underwent combined ACL and PCL reconstructions.[20]

Preoperative Motion Deficits Failure to achieve terminal hyperextension preoperatively results in poor outcomes.[6] In a study by Cosgarea and associates,[17,21] arthrofibrosis occurred in 19% of patients with extension deficits of 10° or more compared with only 8% of patients who had extension deficits of less than 10°.

Surgical Technique Many technical factors have been associated with postoperative motion loss. Nonisometric grafts, graft malposition, and overtensioning of grafts may cause motion loss after ACL surgery.[5,6,22,23] Extra-articular procedures also increase the risk for motion loss. Harner and associates[24] reported that procedures involving the medial capsule, such as medial collateral ligament repair and posterior oblique ligament (MCL) repair, are associated with a higher incidence of motion loss.

Postoperative Rehabilitation Aggressive rehabilitation programs after ACL surgery stress early motion and weight bearing; arthrofibrosis is more likely to develop in patients who have had excessive postoperative immobilization. Cosgarea and associates[17,21] reported that arthrofibrosis developed in 23.4% of patients immobilized at 45° of flexion for 7 days postoperatively, whereas it developed in only 2.7% of patients placed in full extension postoperatively.

Infection Infection also can increase the rate of arthrofibrosis after ACL repair.[5,6,25] The infection enhances the inflammatory process, increases synovitis, and may lead to enhanced recruitment of fibrogenic cytokines. Infection also causes pain that interferes with postoperative rehabilitation and early motion.

Complex Regional Pain Syndrome CRPS or causalgia, which can develop after ACL repair, should be treated aggressively because the pain will affect compliance with postoperative rehabilitation and the prompt return to full ROM. If CRPS is suspected preoperatively, surgery should be postponed.[6]

Management of Arthrofibrosis

General Principles

The treatment of postoperative loss of motion can be tedious and frustrating for the patient, physical therapist, and surgeon. Discussing realistic expectations of both nonsurgical and surgical treatment with patients will help them understand the process and the reasons for additional postoperative rehabilitation.

If a patient has motion loss following an initial ACL reconstruction, a thorough history and physical examination is necessary, and prior surgical reports should be reviewed. Diagnostic imaging studies also are required and helpful. The standard protocol begins with weight-bearing AP, Merchant, long-leg alignment, and bilateral 30° lateral views to assess for patella infera and potential associated heterotopic ossification. MRI may provide useful information in more severe cases of motion loss. When a plateau is reached, or there is progressive symptomatic loss of motion despite aggressive rehabilitation, possible contributing factors such as CRPS or infection should be considered. If CRPS is present, treatment should be initiated before surgical intervention is considered for the motion loss. Surgical intervention for stiffness in a patient with unrecognized CRPS may exacerbate this process. If infection is present, arthroscopic irrigation and débridement are warranted, and motion loss can be addressed simultaneously. Experienced ligament surgeons who defer ACL reconstruction until motion is restored should have a reoperation rate approaching 1% to 2% annually.

Arthroscopic Technique

Surgical débridement typically is performed as an outpatient procedure with the patient under general anesthesia. Positioning involves re-flexing the waist of the operating table, dropping the foot of the bed to leave the surgically treated leg hanging and placing the contralateral limb in a leg holder (**Figure 5**). This position allows full access to and maximum motion of the knee to undergo surgery. A nonsterile tourniquet is applied, and the extremity is prepared and draped in standard fashion.

Six arthroscopic portals may be used for this procedure. Traditionally, the superomedial portal is an outflow portal, the superolateral portal is an

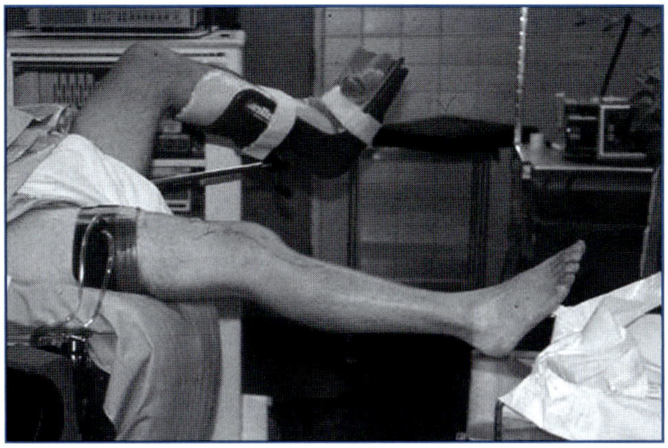

Figure 5 Patient positioning allowing full access to the knee during arthroscopic débridement.

accessory initial viewing portal, the inferolateral portal is the initial arthroscopy portal, and the inferomedial, posteromedial, and posterolateral portals are used as working portals. However, uses for each portal are frequently interchanged based on the specific pathology in any given patient.

Adhesive bands and scar tissue are excised systematically beginning in the suprapatellar pouch (**Figure 6,** *A*). Arthroscopic scissors, basket instruments, shavers, and electrothermal devices are used to débride this area until patellar mobility is restored. The arthroscope is then placed in the superolateral portal, and working instruments are placed in the inferolateral or inferomedial portals to débride the notch and scar tissue extending into the gutters (**Figure 6,** *B*).

Switching the arthroscope back to the inferolateral portal allows further intercondylar notch débridement (**Figure 6,** *C*). At this time a cyclops lesion will be easily visualized if present. Excision of the lesion should follow (**Figure 6,** *D*), with care to avoid débriding the intermeniscal ligament. While débriding in this region it is important to release and mobilize the infrapatellar fat pad from the anterior tibia, thereby reestablishing the pretibial recess and decreasing patellofemoral contact pressures. The arthroscope also should be switched to the inferomedial portal to confirm complete notch débridement, and if present, the sheet of scar tissue extending from the nonarticular margin of the patella also should be removed. Finally, expansion notchplasty may be performed if there is primary graft impingement from notch regrowth.

Anterior joint débridement is completed using the superomedial and inferior portals to address the medial gutter. Motion is then evaluated, and a manipulation may be performed. If motion is still inadequate despite manipulation, we establish the final two portals posteromedially and posterolaterally using an outside-in technique under direct arthroscopic visualization. Once again, particular attention must be paid to avoid neurovascular injury while débriding posteriorly. After scar tissue has been débrided and any loose bodies removed, knee motion is assessed again, and a repeat manipulation can be performed. If motion remains inadequate, an open release as advocated by Cosgarea and associates[17] is likely to be necessary to restore additional motion.

Débriding the intercondylar notch and adjacent anterolateral and anteromedial scar tissue is not the only way to mobilize the patella. We frequently proceed proximally and perform combined medial and lateral releases along with reconstitution of the suprapatellar pouch. Loss of extension generally is attributed to intercondylar notch pathology, whereas loss of flexion usually is secondary to gutter and suprapatellar pouch scar.

When there is significant infrapatellar fat pad scarring, the initial arthroscopy portal may need to be superolateral portal to access the joint and avoid chondral injury with forceful trochar insertion inferiorly. If we cannot easily make a transition into the intercondylar notch and suprapatellar pouch with an inferolateral portal, we use an initial superolateral viewing portal and create an inferomedial working portal to débride the intercondylar notch region first.

Prior to portal closure, meticulous hemostasis is obtained to avoid development of a large hemarthrosis that could compromise gains in ROM. Physical therapy is initiated immediately postoperatively, and a knee immobilizer is prescribed for nighttime use to promote knee extension. An algorithm for the arthroscopic management of arthrofibrosis is outlined in **Figure** 7.

Postoperative Rehabilitation

Millett and associates[25] outlined postoperative rehabilitation of the arthrofibrotic knee, emphasizing

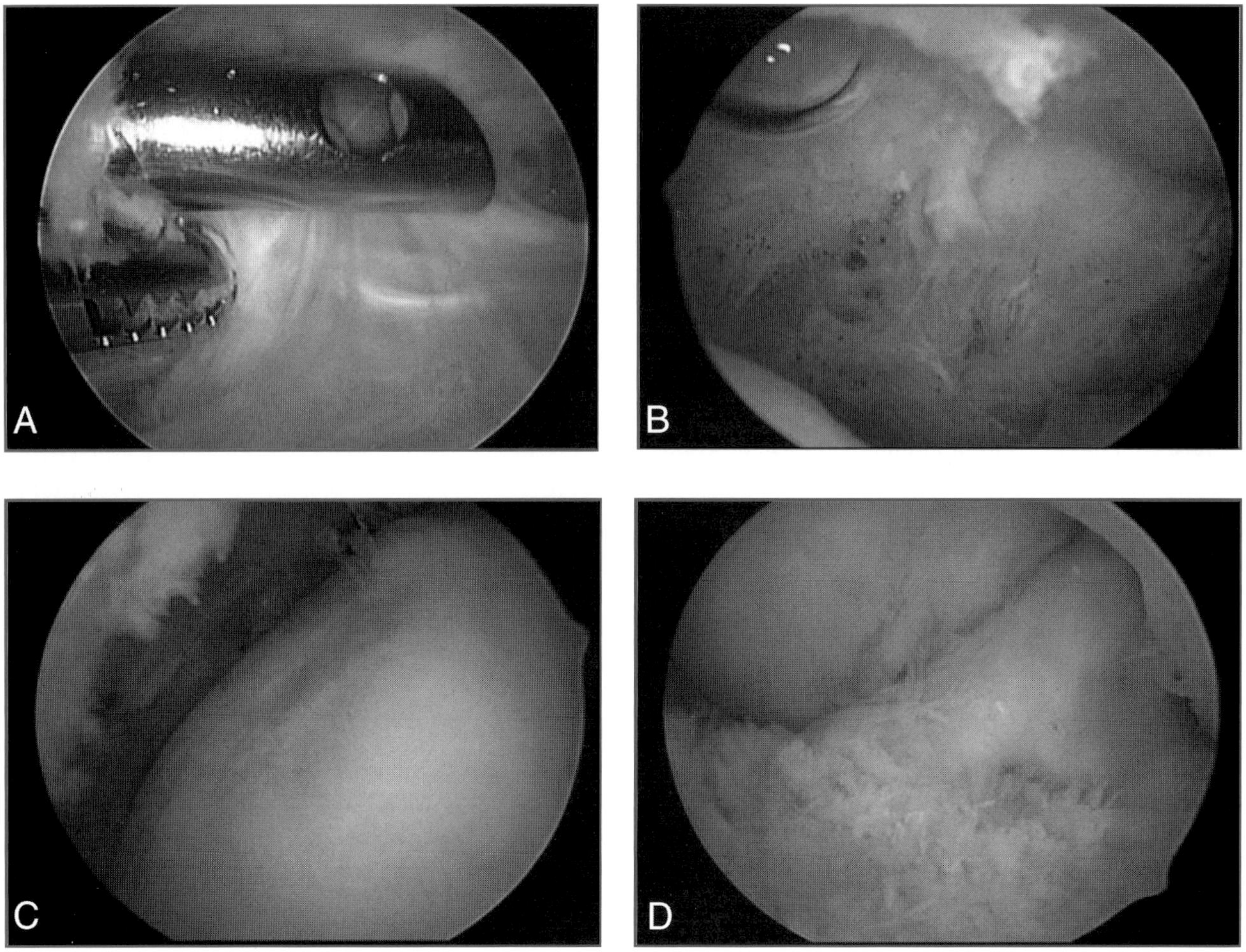

Figure 6 **A,** Débridement of the suprapatellar scar. **B,** After lateral gutter débridement. **C,** Completed anteromedial débridement. **D,** After cyclops resection.

early motion and bracing, if needed, in extension because prolonged immobilization has damaging effects on the joint cartilage, bone, and soft tissue and can lead to motion loss. Flexion contractures usually result from anterior scar formation between the tibia and femur that has developed secondary to immobilization in flexion after surgery;[15] therefore, rehabilitation programs that emphasize early motion and weight bearing will avoid motion problems and result in better overall outcomes.[25]

Two goals to be kept in mind at the conclusion of arthrofibrosis surgery are restoring motion and avoiding damage to the patellar and quadriceps tendons. Passive ROM exercises include seated flexion-extension exercises, prone flexion exercises, heel slides, and wall slides. Patients are encouraged to prop up their heels when resting supine to encourage knee extension. Millett and associates[25] recommend passive ROM four times daily for 15 minutes per session to attain full extension in 2 weeks; the contralateral knee is used as a reference for full extension. Patellar mobility is the most important aspect of rehabilitation, and patellar mobility exercises should be performed with the assistance of a physical therapist in all planes of motion.

Continuous passive motion, bracing, stationary bicycle, treadmill, and aquatherapy can be used as adjuncts. Strengthening exercises should be added after full ROM is attained and there is no swelling, pain, or signs of inflammation. If inflammation

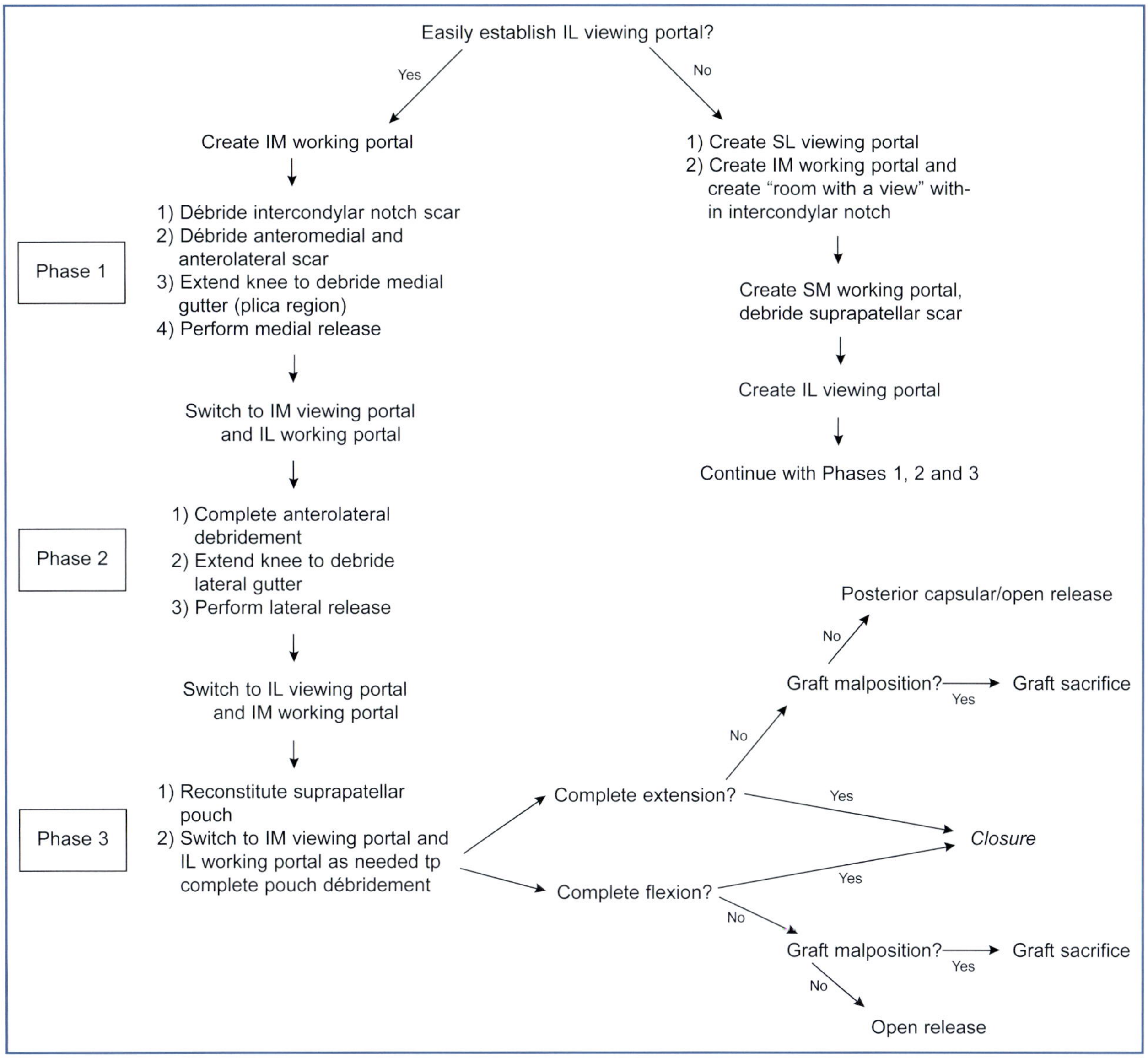

Figure 7 Algorithm for arthroscopic débridement of the stiff knee. (IL = inferolateral, SL = superolateral, IM = inferomedial, SM = superomedial)

develops in the joint, exercises should be discontinued and the inflammation treated aggressively. NSAIDs and analgesics should be used to prevent inflammation and to allow more aggressive rehabilitation.[25]

Patients should be monitored closely after surgery, with frequent communication with the physical therapist or trainer. The typical postoperative course for the patient is prolonged, extending 4 to 6 months before maximum function is restored.

Outcomes

Several authors have reported results of arthroscopic débridement for knee stiffness following ACL reconstruction. Jackson and Schaefer,[11] Marzo and associates,[12] and Fisher and Shelbourne[26] investigated groups of patients with loss of terminal extension and cyclops lesions following ACL reconstruction. They found that débridement yielded good results in most patients, with an average 8° to 12° increase in terminal extension and an average residual flexion contracture of 0° to 4°.

Harner and associates[24] reported on 14 patients who underwent arthroscopic débridement for arthrofibrosis after ACL reconstruction. On average, a 10° improvement in extension was obtained with a residual 3° flexion contracture. Shelbourne and Johnson[15] reported on nine patients who had similar good results following arthroscopic débridement. Eight of the nine patients in this study underwent their index ACL reconstruction within 2 weeks of the initial injury.

Hasan and associates[27] found a symptomatic extension loss greater than 5° in 17 of 342 ACL reconstructions (4%). After arthroscopic débridement (and revision notch plasty in some patients), extension improved an average of 7° and flexion an average of 8°. Despite a small persistent flexion contracture that averaged 3°, there were no significant differences in functional rating scales between this group of patients and a control group of ACL-reconstruction patients who did not have motion loss.

In summary, knee stiffness issues are significantly less frequent or severe than in many of the patients referred to us in the late 1980s and early 1990s. Deferring acute reconstruction until motion is recovered; paying particular attention to combined ACL-MCL injuries; avoiding MCL surgery; staging displaced meniscal repairs, particularly in acute settings; emphasizing complete extension postoperatively; mobilizing the patella; and activating the quadriceps in the immediate postoperative period are some of the many steps that have reduced the severity and frequency of this problem.

Prevention of Arthrofibrosis

Preoperative Evaluation

Acute treatment principles after ACL injury must be followed to minimize the chance of postoperative motion loss. Anti-inflammatory modalities including NSAIDs and ice should be used to minimize swelling and pain. Their use facilitates immediate physical therapy focusing on restoration of knee ROM, particularly terminal hyperextension. Maintaining or reactivating the thigh musculature via quadriceps setting, straight-leg raises, and closed chain exercises also should be stressed. Open chain exercises should be avoided because they are reported to contribute to patellofemoral symptoms in many patients.[28] Finally, activities should be modified to prevent further injury.

The inflammatory phase generally resolves within 1 to 3 weeks, and if pain and swelling do not resolve or if ROM is not restored, a displaced torn meniscus or other mechanical block (loose osteochondral fragments or an incarcerated ACL stump) should be suspected. If present, these extension blocks may need initial arthroscopic treatment and staged ACL reconstruction if there is more than 5° of fixed flexion; loss of more than 5° of terminal extension prior to ACL reconstruction has been shown to correlate with ultimate motion loss.[29]

Timing of Surgery

For acute ACL injuries, the timing of ligament reconstruction remains controversial. In some studies, early reconstruction has been associated with an increased incidence of arthrofibrosis and postoperative motion loss.[24] Compared with recovery after reconstruction in subacute or chronic cases, Wasilewski and associates[30] discovered that patients who underwent early reconstruction had slower recovery of quadriceps strength, higher rates of arthrofibrosis, and slower return of postoperative motion at 3, 6, 12, and 18 months. Furthermore, a faster return of quadriceps strength and a decreased incidence of motion loss are reported when surgery is delayed until initial inflammation subsides and motion is restored.[17] Therefore, many authors recommend waiting 3 to 4 weeks after the injury before proceeding with ACL reconstruction.[16,24] Others believe that there is no absolute period of time in which surgery should be delayed and, when using an aggressive postoperative physical therapy protocol, have not reported significant complications with early ACL reconstruction. However, in the study by Hunter and associates,[31] all patients who required reoperation for motion loss had had reconstructive surgery within 2 weeks of the injury.

Unfortunately, the lack of uniformity among patient selection, surgical technique, postoperative rehabilitation protocol, and follow-up data makes it difficult to synthesize the results of these and other relevant case series. However, we recommend deferring ACL reconstruction until inflammation has subsided and knee motion is normal to near normal. Restoration of the last few degrees of extension or hyperextension may be difficult if a stump of torn ACL is incarcerated in the anterolateral joint. Symmetric flexion usually is regained easily unless there is an associated MCL sprain. Robins and associates[32] discussed the anatomic location of an MCL injury and how it may impact motion recovery. These authors observed that proximal MCL injuries are more problematic and can contribute to slower recovery of full flexion. With isolated ACL injuries, our patients frequently regain 95% to 100% of preoperative ROM within 4 weeks; therefore, we agree with the recommendation of Harner and associates[24] and others who advocate waiting 3 to 4 weeks after the injury before performing ACL reconstruction. This common sense approach separates initial posttraumatic inflammation from postoperative inflammation.

Graft Selection

Extensor mechanism complications are more commonly reported with patellar tendon autografts than with other graft sources, partially because of their popularity (eg, versus quadriceps tendon grafts, which have not attained universal acceptance or popularity). Certainly patellar fractures and patellar tendon ruptures are exclusive to extensor mechanism harvest. However, loss of motion and anterior knee pain occur after both patellar tendon and hamstring ACL reconstructions. Freedman and associates[33] performed a meta-analysis of studies with a minimum 24-month follow-up comparing ACL reconstruction with patellar tendon and hamstrings autografts. The patellar tendon group had a higher rate of manipulation under anesthesia or lysis of adhesions for symptomatic loss of motion (6% versus 3%) and of anterior knee pain (17% versus 11%). It is unclear whether the higher prevalence of these complications in patients with patellar tendon autografts is a result of the trauma of graft harvest or simply of differences in postoperative rehabilitation between these two patient groups.

Intraoperative Factors

Many technical factors at the time of reconstruction also have been associated with ultimate motion loss and secondary anterior knee pain. One of the most common avoidable causes of postoperative stiffness is graft malposition. A tibial or femoral tunnel that is placed too far anterior or failure to perform an adequate notchplasty can lead to graft-notch impingement, resulting in a primary block to extension. A nonisometric anterior graft also will interfere with normal knee kinematics and secondarily limit flexion or elongate to accommodate increased flexion angles.[34,35]

Whether excessive tension in the ACL graft leads to loss of motion is controversial. Some authors believe that if the graft is properly positioned, its natural viscoelastic properties will accommodate excessive tension and allow full knee ROM without graft failure.[36] Others believe that if a graft is too tight, eg, not fixed with the knee in full extension, biomechanics dictate that there will be increased strain on knee extension and the graft will either limit terminal extension or stretch during early rehabilitative efforts to regain extension.[37] Currently, the best initial tension and knee position at the time of graft fixation remains debatable. We recommend fixing the graft in complete extension or hyperextension, with the knee axially loaded and with very firm tension applied to the graft.

Postoperative Rehabilitation

Historically, rehabilitation protocols have avoided early extension exercises and weight bearing for fear of excessive graft strain and loss of knee stability.[38] However, Rubinstein and associates[39] and Shelbourne and associates[16] have reported similar KT-1000 arthrometer side-to-side manual maximum stability when comparing patients who achieved early full hyperextension with those who did not. Furthermore, motion loss and anterior knee pain have been associated with less aggressive protocols.

Contemporary postoperative rehabilitation programs emphasize patellar mobilization and

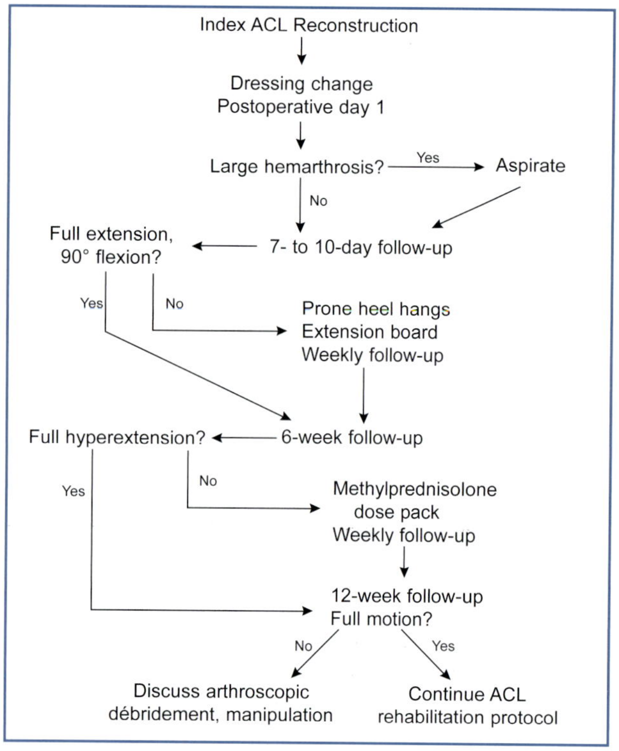

Figure 8 Algorithm for postoperative motion recovery.

immediate full passive extension combined with night extension bracing. Early active extension, straight-leg raises, closed kinetic chain exercises, and immediate weight bearing in extension are allowed to promote early muscle control and quadriceps reactivation. ROM is carefully monitored to identify knees at risk for postoperative motion loss. Initial goals include full extension to 90° of flexion within the first 2 weeks. For problematic extension initially, prone heel hangs with or without weights can be added. Judicious use of cryotherapy, NSAIDs, electrical stimulation, iontophoresis, and phonophoresis can be helpful. In cases of prolonged postoperative inflammation, methylprednisolone dose packs occasionally are used at 6 weeks postoperatively. By focusing on early motion and weight bearing, extension is restored more quickly, and a lower incidence of late motion problems and anterior knee pain can be expected.[40] Failure to achieve terminal hyperextension, either because of a suboptimal rehabilitation protocol or an unmotivated patient, will likely result in a poor clinical outcome. Our algorithm for postoperative motion recovery is outlined in **Figure 8**.

Management and Outcome Summary

The patient's knee was débrided using four anterior portals and the systematic approach previously described. Following débridement, examination and gentle manipulation yielded 2° of terminal hyperextension, equaling that of the contralateral knee. Normal patellar mobility was also observed intraoperatively after débridement.

Postoperatively, the patient was given a knee immobilizer to promote nighttime extension. Physical therapy was initiated with a focus on prone heel hangs, use of a knee extension board, and closed chain quadriceps exercises to maintain terminal hyperextension. At follow-up, the patient had recovered symmetric hyperextension and symmetric patellar mobility, and his anterior knee pain had resolved.

Strategies to Minimize Common Complications

Because the results of surgery for arthrofibrosis are only fair, prevention is preferred. Surgery should be delayed until signs of local inflammation have abated. The knee should not have a significant effusion, and full ROM should be achieved before surgery. Preoperative physical therapy is helpful to restore muscle strength and ROM before surgery, and it may facilitate the postoperative recovery as well. NSAIDs also may be of benefit in decreasing the inflammatory response that follows ACL injury.

Technical errors, such as malpositioned or overtensioned grafts are a common source of postoperative motion loss with resultant arthrofibrosis. Because the results with revision surgery are inferior to primary procedures, careful attention to the technical aspects of ACL reconstruction is essential.

Postoperative physical therapy programs that emphasize early motion, particularly passive and active extension, are especially important in preventing postoperative motion loss. Bracing the knee in extension is also important because the loss of extension is much more poorly tolerated than any loss of flexion.

References

1. Ferrari JD, Bush-Joseph CA, Bach BR Jr: Endoscopic anterior cruciate ligament reconstruction with patellar tendon autograft: Surgical technique. *Tech Orthop* 1998;13:262-274.
2. Strum GM, Friedman MJ, Fox JM, et al: Acute anterior cruciate ligament reconstruction: Analysis of complications. *Clin Orthop* 1990;253:184-189.
3. DeCarlo MS, Sell K: Normative data for range of motion and single leg hop in high school athletes. *J Sports Rehabil* 1997;6:246-255.
4. Benum P: Operative mobilization of stiff knees after surgical treatment of knee injuries and post-traumatic conditions. *Acta Orthop Scand* 1982;53:625-631.
5. Millett PJ, Wickiewicz TL, Warren RF: Motion loss after ligament injuries to the knee: Part II. Prevention and treatment. *Am J Sports Med* 2001;29:822-828.
6. DeHaven KE, Cosgarea AJ, Sebastianelli WJ: Arthrofibrosis of the knee following ligament surgery. *Instr Course Lect* 2003;52:369-381.
7. Shelbourne KD, Patel DV, Martini DJ: Classification and management of arthrofibrosis of the knee after anterior cruciate ligament surgery. *Am J Sports Med* 1996;24:857-862.
8. Paulos LE, Rosenberg TD, Drawbert J, et al: Infrapatellar contracture syndrome: An unrecognized cause of knee stiffness with patella entrapment and patella infera. *Am J Sports Med* 1987;15:331-341.
9. Ahmad CS, Kwak SD, Ateshian GA, et al: Effects of patellar tendon adhesion to the anterior tibia on knee mechanics. *Am J Sports Med* 1998;26:715-724.
10. Paulos LE, Wnorowski DC, Greenwald AE: Infrapatellar contracture syndrome: Diagnosis, treatment, and long-term follow-up. *Am J Sports Med* 1994;22:440-449.
11. Jackson DW, Schaefer RK: Cyclops syndrome: Loss of extension following intra-articular anterior cruciate ligament reconstruction. *Arthroscopy* 1990;6:171-178.
12. Marzo JM, Bowen MK, Warren RF, et al: Intraarticular fibrous nodule as a cause of loss of extension following anterior cruciate ligament reconstruction. *Arthroscopy* 1992;8:10-18.
13. Delincé P, Krallis P, Descamps PY, et al: Different aspects of the cyclops lesion following anterior cruciate ligament reconstruction: A multifactorial etiopathogenesis. *Arthroscopy* 1998;14:869-876.
14. Shelbourne KD, Trumper RV: Preventing anterior knee pain after anterior cruciate ligament reconstruction. *Am J Sports Med* 1997;25:41-47.
15. Shelbourne KD, Johnson GE: The outpatient surgical management of arthrofibrosis after anterior cruciate ligament surgery. *Am J Sports Med* 1994;22:192-197.
16. Shelbourne KD, Wilckens JH, Mollabashy A, et al: Arthrofibrosis in acute anterior cruciate ligament reconstruction. *Am J Sports Med* 1991;19:332-336.
17. Cosgarea AJ, Sebastianelli WJ, DeHaven KE: Prevention of arthrofibrosis after anterior cruciate ligament reconstruction using the central third patellar tendon autograft. *Am J Sports Med* 1995;23:87-92.
18. Nogalski MP: A review of early anterior cruciate ligament surgical repair or reconstruction: Results and caveats. *Orthop Rev* 1993;22:1213-1223.
19. Shapiro MS, Freedman EL: Allograft reconstruction of the anterior and posterior cruciate ligaments after traumatic knee dislocation. *Am J Sports Med* 1995;23:580-587
20. Sisto DJ, Warren RF: Complete knee dislocation: A follow-up study of operative treatment. *Clin Orthop* 1985;198:94-101.
21. Cosgarea AJ, DeHaven KE, Lovelock JE: The surgical treatment of arthrofibrosis of the knee. *Am J Sports Med* 1994;22:184-191.
22. Eakin C: Knee arthrofibrosis: Prevention and management of a potentially devastating condition. *Physician Sports Med* 2001;29:822-828.
23. Romano VM, Graf BK, Keene JS, et al: Anterior cruciate ligament reconstruction: The effect of tibial tunnel placement on range of motion. *Am J Sports Med* 1993;21:415-418.
24. Harner CD, Irrgang JJ, Paul J, et al: Loss of motion after anterior cruciate ligament reconstruction. *Am J Sports Med* 1992;20:499-506.
25. Millett PJ, Johnson B, Carlson J, Krishnan S, Steadman JR: Rehabilitation of the arthrofibrotic knee. *Am J Orthop* 2003;32:531-538.
26. Fisher SE, Shelbourne KD: Arthroscopic treatment of symptomatic extension block complicating anterior cruciate ligament reconstruction. *Am J Sports Med* 1993;2:558-564.
27. Hasan SS, Saleem A, Bach BR Jr, et al: Results of arthroscopic treatment of symptomatic loss of extension following anterior cruciate ligament reconstruction. *Am J Knee Surg* 2000;13:201-292.
28. Grood ES, Suntay WJ, Noyes FR, et al: Biomechanics of knee extension exercise. *J Bone Joint Surg Am* 1984;66:725-734.

29. McHugh MP, Tyler TF, Gleim GW, et al: Preoperative indicators of motion loss and weakness following anterior cruciate ligament reconstruction. *J Orthop Sports Phys Ther* 1998;27:407-411.

30. Wasilewski SA, Covall DJ, Cohen S: Effect of surgical timing on recovery and associated injuries after anterior cruciate ligament reconstruction. *Am J Sports Med* 1993;21:338-342.

31. Hunter RE, Mastrangelo J, Freeman JR, et al: The impact of surgical timing on postoperative motion and stability following anterior cruciate ligament reconstruction. *Arthroscopy* 1996;12:667-674.

32. Robins AJ, Newman AP, Burks RT: Postoperative return of motion in anterior cruciate ligament and medial collateral ligament injuries: The effect of medial collateral ligament rupture location. *Am J Sports Med* 1993;21:20-25.

33. Freedman KB, D'Amato MJ, Nedeff DD, Kaz A, Bach BR Jr: Arthroscopic anterior cruciate ligament reconstruction: A meta-analysis comparing patellar tendon and hamstring tendon autografts. *Am J Sports Med* 2003;31:2-11.

34. Fu FH, Bennett CH, Ma CB, et al: Current trends in anterior cruciate ligament reconstruction: Part II. Operative procedures and clinical correlations. *Am J Sports Med* 2000;28:124-130.

35. Yaru NC, Daniel DM, Penner D: The effect of tibial attachment site on graft impingement in an anterior cruciate ligament reconstruction. *Am J Sports Med* 1992;20:217-220.

36. Millett PJ, Wickiewicz TL, Warren RF: Motion loss after ligament injuries to the knee: Part I. Causes. *Am J Sports Med* 2001;29:664-675.

37. Nabors ED, Richmond JC, Vannah WM, et al: Anterior cruciate ligament graft tensioning in full extension. *Am J Sports Med* 1995;23:488-492.

38. Paulos L, Noyes FR, Good E, et al: Knee rehabilitation after anterior cruciate ligament reconstruction and repair. *Am J Sports Med* 1981;9:140-149.

39. Rubinstein RA Jr, Shelbourne KD, VanMeter CD, et al: Effect on knee stability if full hyperextension is restored immediately after autogenous bone-patellar-bone anterior cruciate ligament reconstruction. *Am J Sports Med* 1995;23:365-368.

40. Noyes FR, Mangine RE, Barber SD: The early treatment of motion complications after reconstruction of the anterior cruciate ligament. *Clin Orthop* 1993;277:217-228.

Chapter 6

Failed ACL Reconstruction: Evaluation for Revision ACL Reconstruction

Mitchell Fagelman, MD
Kevin B. Freedman, MD, MSCE

Case Presentation

History

A 26-year-old man sustained a twisting injury to his right knee while playing football 10 years ago. He sought medical attention for right knee pain and instability within 2 weeks of the injury. Examination at that time revealed a large effusion, a grade IIB Lachman test, and medial joint line tenderness. MRI scans obtained at that time revealed an acute anterior cruciate ligament (ACL) tear and a large bucket-handle medial meniscus tear (**Figure 1**). After all treatment options were discussed, the patient elected to undergo a bone-patellar tendon-bone (BTB) autograft ACL reconstruction and a partial meniscectomy (**Figure 2**). Extensive physical therapy followed.

Current Problem and Treatment

Three years after surgery, the patient sustained a second twisting injury to the same knee. Since that time, he has had recurrent instability with any planting or twisting activities. He also has had pain, predominantly on the medial side of the knee, which is exacerbated by the episodes of instability, and pain and stiffness with prolonged standing. He had not had physical therapy since the second injury. After 2 years of persistent and increasing pain, resulting in decreased activity with the knee, the patient presented for examination.

Physical examination at this time revealed that the patient walked with a normal gait and had normal knee alignment. Both the patellar harvest scar and lateral incision appeared well healed. The patient's range of motion (ROM) was from 0° to 130°, and he had medial joint line tenderness but no lateral-sided tenderness, no significant patellofemoral crepitus, and negative patellar grind and patellar inhibition testing. Ligament testing revealed a grade IIIB+ Lachman test, a positive pivot-shift test, but no concomitant laxity.

AP and lateral radiographs obtained at this time showed the appropriate position of interference screws consistent with a two-incision ACL reconstruction (**Figure 3**) and no significant osteoarthritis. MRI of his right knee revealed a complete tear of the ACL graft and a complex tear of the medial meniscus with nearly complete absence of the posterior horn of the medial meniscus (**Figure 4**).

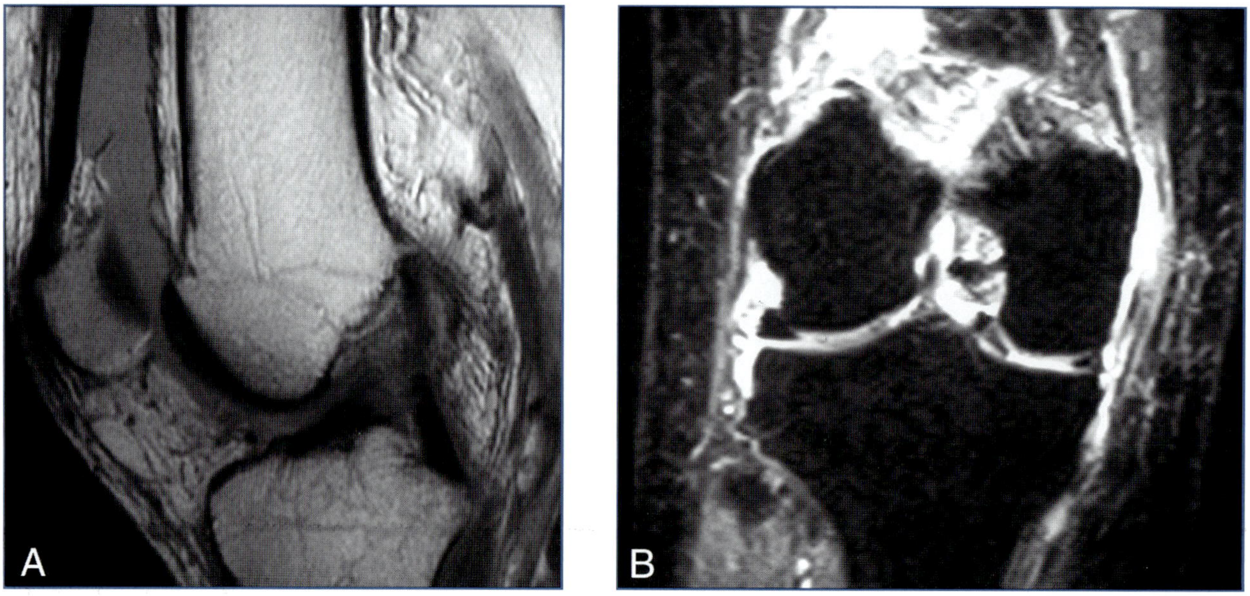

Figure 1 **A,** Sagittal T1-weighted MRI scan showing an acute ACL tear. **B,** Coronal T2-weighted MRI scan showing a displaced bucket-handle meniscus tear.

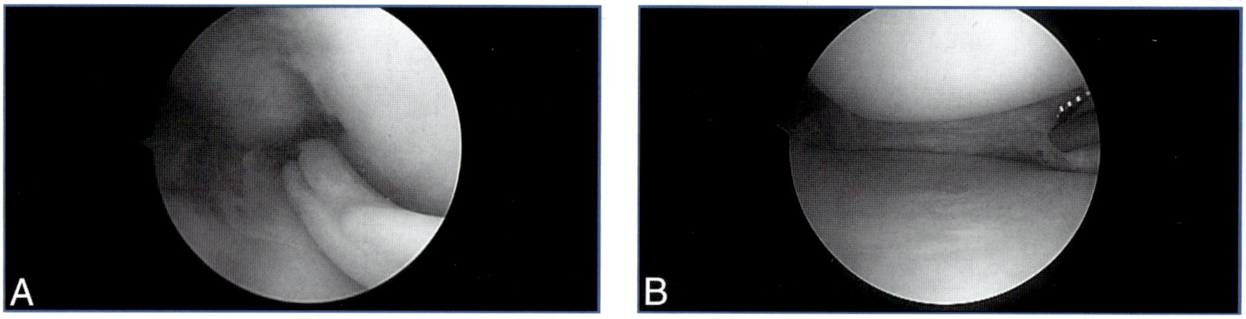

Figure 2 **A,** Arthroscopic image showing a displaced bucket-handle fragment of the medial meniscus in the intercondylar notch. **B,** Arthroscopic image of the medial compartment following resection of the bucket-handle fragment with partial meniscectomy.

The patient's clinical presentation and imaging studies suggest ACL insufficiency following reconstruction and medial meniscus deficiency. The failure was attributed to repeat trauma combined with secondary laxity from meniscal deficiency. Given the patient's degree of instability and his activity level, revision ACL reconstruction was recommended. In addition, because of the meniscal deficiency and loss of the secondary stabilizer to anterior tibial translation, a concomitant meniscus transplant was indicated.

Discussion

Recognizing the Problem

Failure of primary ACL reconstruction has been attributed to three principal causes: technical errors, biologic failures, and traumatic failures.[1-5] A secondary cause is failure to recognize or address associated laxity at the time of primary ACL reconstruction.[6,7] Failure can be caused by

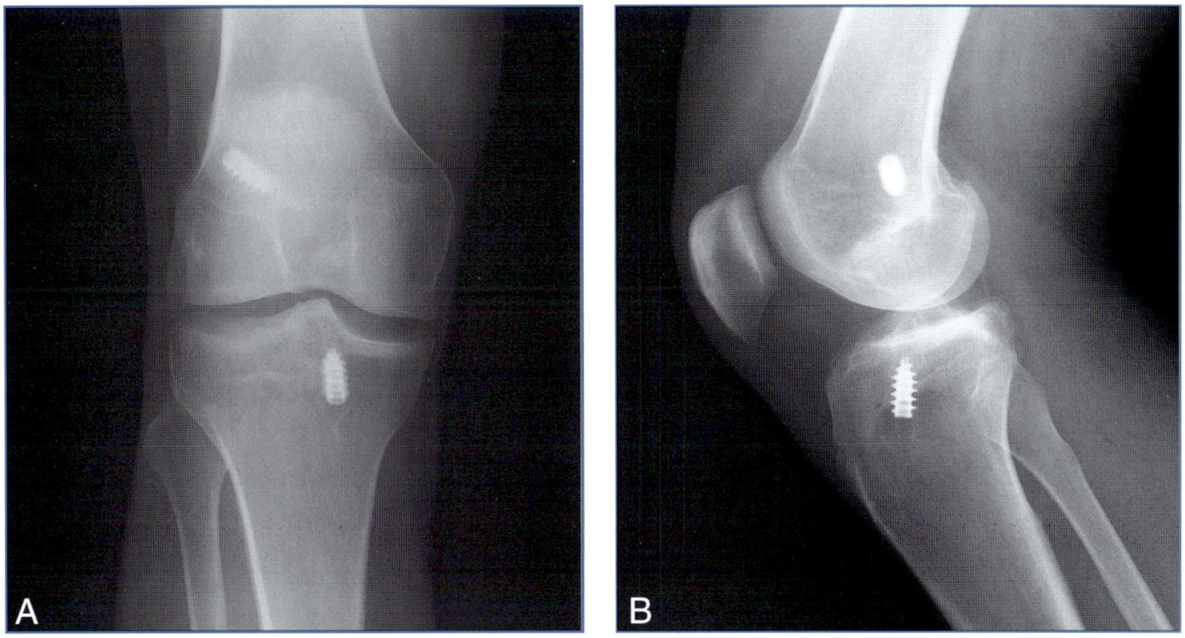

Figure 3 AP **(A)** and lateral **(B)** radiographs showing a two-incision ACL reconstruction with metal interference screws in place. Note that the tunnels are appropriately placed.

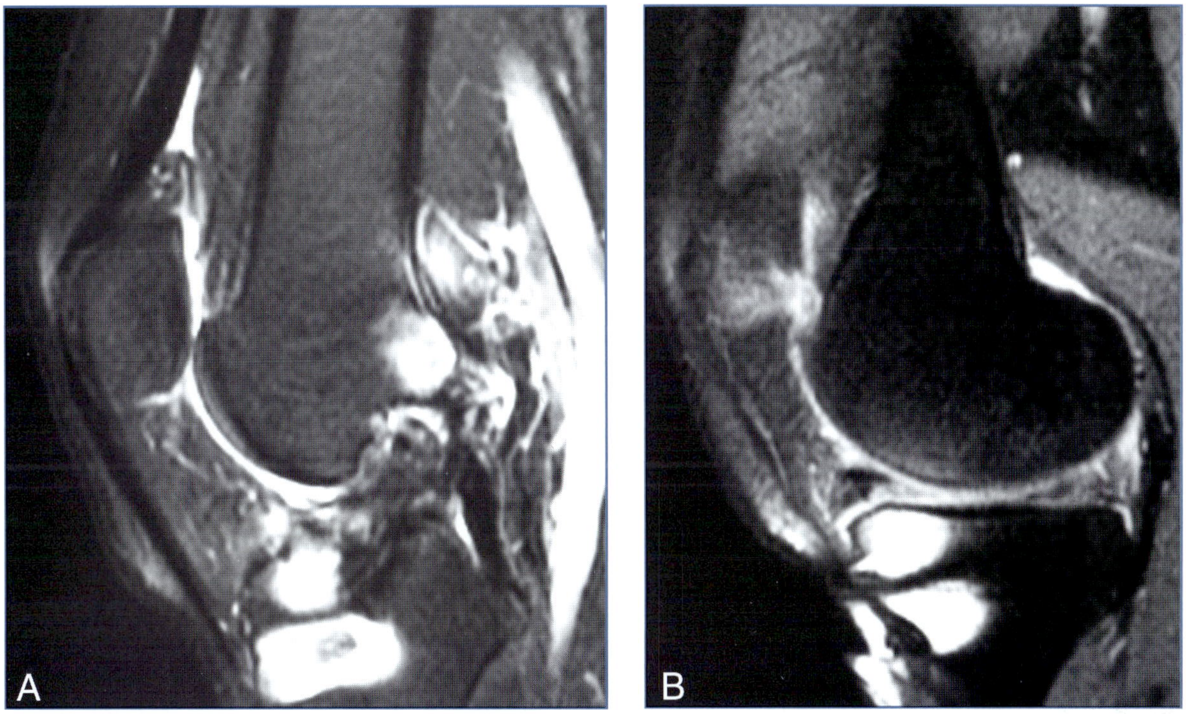

Figure 4 Sagittal T2-weighted MRI scans showing a chronic ACL tear following reconstruction **(A)** and near complete absence of the posterior horn of the medial meniscus following partial medial meniscectomy **(B)**.

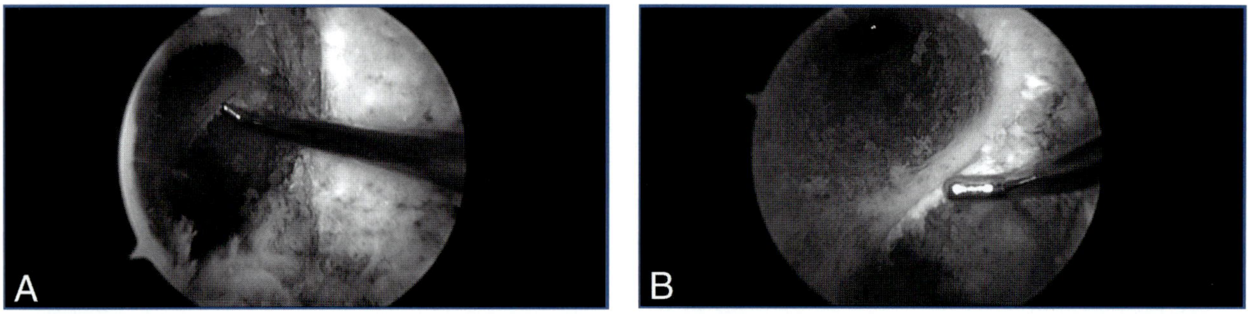

Figure 5 **A,** Arthroscopic image of a right knee showing the appropriate femoral tunnel position. The socket is placed at the 10:30 position within 1 to 2 mm of the back wall of the intercondylar notch. **B,** Close-up image of the femoral socket showing that only 1 to 2 mm of posterior wall remains to ensure that the tunnel is positioned as far posteriorly as possible.

one or more of these factors in isolation or in combination.

The source of failure must be identified before a revision procedure in an effort to prevent repeating previous errors and to help formulate an organized, systematic plan for any future surgery. Failures can be classified according to when they occur. Early failures occur within the first 6 months after surgery and are most often a result of poor surgical technique, failure of graft incorporation, or overly aggressive rehabilitation. Late failures occur more than 1 year after surgery and usually result from a repeat traumatic injury.

Technical Errors

Technical errors account for most failed ACL reconstructions[8-12] and include improper tunnel placement (most common), improper graft tensioning, inadequate notchplasty, and inadequate graft fixation. These issues are briefly described here, but in more detail in chapter 7.

Improper Tunnel Placement Improper tunnel placement causes 70% to 80% of failed ACL reconstructions.[5,11-13] The most common error, improper position of the femoral tunnel, often is caused by poor visualization during surgery.[2,8,14] Therefore, adequate visualization is critical before drilling either the femoral or tibial tunnels. Traditionally, a correctly placed femoral tunnel originates at the 1 to 1:30 o'clock position in the left knee and the 10:30 to 11 o'clock position in the right knee in the coronal plane. In the sagittal plane, only 1 to 2 mm of posterior cortical shell in the over-the-top position can offer near-anatomic tunnel position[15] (**Figure 5**).

Because the native ACL can accommodate only minimal changes in length before undergoing plastic deformation and stretching, placing an ACL graft outside the anatomic position can cause undue stress and graft failure. If the femoral tunnel is placed too far anterior, the graft will be placed under excessive tension during flexion, leading to decreased flexion or stretching of the graft. If the tunnel is placed too far posterior, posterior wall blowout may occur. A vertically placed femoral tunnel may not prevent persistent rotational instability (**Figure 6,** *A*). Although the anterior-posterior translation can be corrected (with a normalized Lachman), the knee may pivot around a vertical graft.[16] Finally, a misplaced femoral tunnel in the coronal plane may cause impingement on the lateral femoral condyle or the posterior cruciate ligament (PCL) (**Figure 6,** *B*).

A poorly placed tibial tunnel is less common, but it also can result in graft failure. A tunnel placed too anterior can lead to notch impingement and a lack of extension, and a tunnel placed too posterior can lead to instability in flexion. Because the position of the tibial tunnel dictates placement of the femoral tunnel, correct placement of the tibial tunnel is crucial. The tibial tunnel ideally is located 7 to 8 mm anterior to the PCL and parallel to the posterior aspect of the anterior horn of the lateral meniscus[17] (**Figure 7**). The footprint of the torn ACL also may help ensure proper pin positioning before reaming.

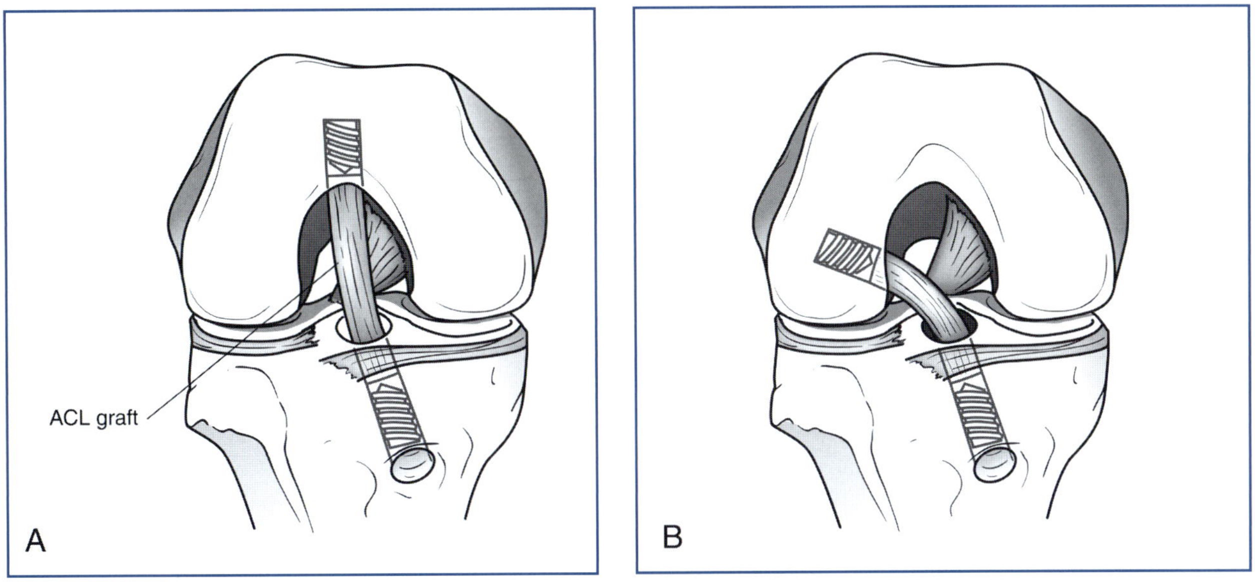

Figure 6 Illustrations of a right knee in which the femoral tunnel is improperly placed. A tunnel placed too vertically **(A)** can cause impingement of the ACL graft on the PCL, whereas a tunnel placed too laterally **(B)** can cause impingement of the graft on the lateral femoral condyle.

Improper Graft Tensioning Neither the optimal tensioning of the ACL graft nor the definitive angle of the knee during graft tensioning is known. However, many authors recommend flexing the knee between 15° and 30° while tensioning the graft.[9,15,18-20] Cycling the graft through a normal ROM and holding tension until graft fixation also may help prevent stress-relaxation of the graft,[21] and performing a Lachman test while visualizing the graft arthroscopically will confirm adequate tension after fixation.[15]

Factors that influence the overall graft tension include type of graft material, tunnel placement, physiologic joint laxity, and knee angle at the time of fixation. Excessive tensioning of the graft can lead to decreased motion, mucoid degeneration of the graft, delayed vascularization, graft failure, and possibly osteoarthritis.[10,21,22] In contrast, undertensioning the graft could lead to excess knee laxity.

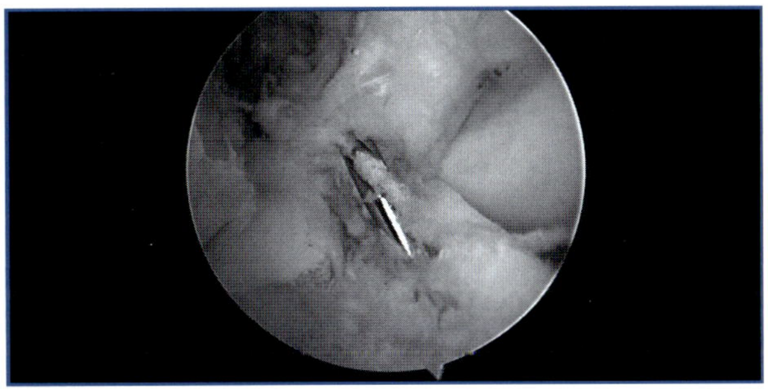

Figure 7 Arthroscopic image showing the tibial guide pin placed before reaming of the tibial tunnel. The tunnel is in the posterior aspect of the ACL footprint in the center of the intercondylar notch, approximately 7 mm anterior to the PCL and parallel to the posterior aspect of the anterior horn of the lateral meniscus.

Graft Impingement Performing an adequate notchplasty without removing too much bone is critical to the success of ACL reconstruction. Without an adequate notchplasty, graft impingement in extension can occur, leading to repetitive trauma to the graft and subsequent failure. However, overly aggressive notchplasty must be avoided to help prevent improper placement of the femoral tunnel and ensure adequate bone stock for fixation.[23,24] Some authors advocate removing sufficient bone to allow the posterior horn of the lateral meniscus to be visualized through the notch.[9]

Overall, the most important aspect of notchplasty is adequate visualization of the posterior wall and the over-the-top position.

MRI can be used to assess for impingement of the graft in failed primary ACL reconstructions.[3] Mixed MRI signals are found in graft impingement in contrast to the homogenous signal found in grafts that are normal.[14] These MRI changes are time dependent and typically well established within 3 months after surgery.

Failure of Graft Fixation Because early and aggressive postoperative ROM exercises are crucial to a good outcome in revision ACL surgery, secure graft fixation is vital to prevent changes in position within the tunnels until graft incorporation occurs. Various types of fixation devices are available, and the overall strength of fixation depends on bone density, the integrity and size of the tunnels, the type of graft, and the method of fixation.[25,26] Improper screw size, divergent or convergent tunnels, and/or laceration of tensioning sutures are all possible impediments to adequate graft fixation. Whatever method of fixation is chosen, careful surgical technique is paramount to obtain a strong ACL graft that is able to withstand a rigorous postoperative protocol.

Biologic Failure

Biologic failure should be suspected in patients with persistent instability but no history of trauma and after technical error has been ruled out.[8] All grafts used for ACL reconstruction differ biologically from the native ACL. Tendon grafts differ in fiber length and orientation, vascular supply, and fibroblast activity.[27] Inadequate vascularity, immunologic responses to allograft, and stress shielding by implants are potential sources of intrinsic graft failure reported in animal studies.[2,28-31] Graft incorporation has been reported to take as long as 12 weeks in an animal model.[32]

Infection and arthrofibrosis are other potential causes of biologic graft failure.[6,33,34] Postoperative infection is rare but can be devastating. Williams and associates[34] reported a 0.3% infection rate in arthroscopically assisted ACL surgeries. Removal of the graft was necessary in four of seven patients. Arthrofibrosis following ACL reconstruction is also a dreadful complication that is associated with a number of factors, including inadequate preoperative motion, intraoperative technical errors, and inadequate postoperative rehabilitation.[35] Prevention of arthrofibrosis is essential because this postoperative loss of motion can be more distressing to the patient than the preoperative instability that necessitated the ACL reconstruction.

Traumatic Failure

If a thorough history, physical examination, and radiographic evaluation do not identify the reason for failed ACL reconstruction, it can be assumed that the ACL graft was stable and functional before reinjury. In the athletic population, between 5% and 10% of failures are caused by trauma.[13] Traumatic failure has been divided into two broad categories:[8] early failure before graft incorporation and late failure (after 6 months) following complete rehabilitation. Overaggressive rehabilitation, patient noncompliance, significant traumatic reinjury, and premature return to sports are possible causes of early traumatic failure. Biomechanical studies report that during the first postoperative year the stiffness of allograft or autograft tendons is less than 50% that of control subjects, a clear indication that grafts are more prone to traumatic failure.[28] Bone-to-bone healing may take 6 weeks, whereas bone-to-tendon healing may take up to 8 to 12 weeks. Late failure usually occurs as a result of a significant traumatic injury to a stable knee. Often this traumatic reinjury is followed by an immediate knee effusion, which can be a helpful sign during initial physical examination.

Associated Ligament Deficiencies

Posterolateral instability is perhaps the most common unrecognized and untreated ligament deficiency associated with revision ACL reconstruction. Failure to recognize associated ligament deficiencies before ACL reconstruction results in chronic repetitive microtrauma, causing increased forces on the ACL graft. Noyes and Barber-Westin[36] reported that 31% of their patients with ACL reconstructions had either unrecognized or untreated lateral, posterolateral, or medial ligament deficiency at the time of revision surgery. Examination of the ACL-posterolateral complex consists of a Lachman test at 30° of flexion and a dial test. Posterolateral instability is defined here as at least 10° of increased tibial external rotation in the affected knee compared with the normal knee at 30° of flexion. If the posterolateral complex is abnormal, surgical options include primary repair, and/or advancement or recession, along with augmentation or reconstruction of the lateral collateral ligament, popliteofibular tendon, and/or popliteal tendon.

Because the posterior horn of the medial meniscus provides stability in an ACL-deficient knee, patients with a previous meniscectomy may have secondary laxity. Partial or complete absence of the meniscus alters joint kinematics and can lead to abnormal forces on the graft. Combining ACL reconstruction with medial meniscal transplant is controversial but may restore anterior-posterior knee stability following ACL reconstruction. Young ACL-deficient patients with instability and focal compartmental symptoms after partial or complete meniscectomy may be the best candidates for this combined procedure. Harner and associates[2] reported that 82% of their patients who underwent concurrent revision ACL reconstruction and medial meniscus transplant improved after surgery, with 90% rating their level of function as normal or nearly normal.

Varus alignment of the knee also can place undue stress on the ACL graft and cause reconstruction failure. Noyes and associates[37] advocate a high tibial osteotomy for ACL-deficient knees with significant varus. They reported that 80% of their patients maintained their correction in these complex knee injuries. Thus, the surgeon must determine whether a staged procedure should be used to correct both varus alignment and ACL deficiency. If the patient has varus alignment with abnormal lateral joint line opening and varus thrust on gait, high tibial osteotomy should be performed first and ACL revision later.[36]

Managing the Problem

Preoperative Evaluation

Because revision ACL reconstructions are complex, a detailed understanding of the patient's history is more critical at this time than before the index procedure. The following questions must be answered: (1) Did the primary procedure alleviate the initial symptoms? (2) Are the current symptoms similar to or different from symptoms before the index procedure? (3) Is pain constant, does it occur during daily activities, or does it occur only during rigorous activity? (4) What was the postoperative rehabilitation, and did the patient comply with this protocol?

A thorough physical examination is essential and must focus on ligamentous and meniscal structures, as well as overall axial alignment of the leg. In addition to confirming an ACL deficiency, the examination should focus on other possible intra-articular pathology or concomitant problems. Joint line tenderness or recurrent effusion may suggest meniscal pathology. Prior skin incisions should be noted and potential wound healing problems addressed. Ligament testing should evaluate the integrity of the ACL and PCL, as well as any varus-valgus laxity. Careful examination of the posterolateral structures for associated ligament deficiency is crucial but often overlooked. Knee ROM is an important indicator of residual flexion contractures, arthrofibrosis, or extensor mechanism dysfunction. In addition, patellar mobility and the presence of any patellofemoral degeneration such as crepitus must be assessed. These considerations are important, especially if the surgeon is considering harvesting a BTB or quadriceps-bone-tendon graft. Examination of gait for a varus thrust is valuable because this problem also may require surgical intervention, either before or in combination with revision ACL reconstruction, as previously mentioned.

Several other key pieces of information are needed for a comprehensive preoperative evaluation of the knee. Prior medical records, including surgical reports and arthroscopic photographs, are important to review while planning for surgery. Radiographs, including standard AP and lateral views, weight-bearing 45° flexion PA views, Merchant views, and/or long-cassette mechanical axis views, can be used to assess lower extremity alignment, tunnel position, and location of hardware. MRI can be useful to evaluate graft integrity and other associated pathology, including meniscal lesions and articular cartilage damage. The combination of plain radiographs and MRI usually provides sufficient information for preoperative planning for revision ACL reconstruction. These imaging studies provide the necessary information regarding tunnel position and subchondral bony changes, chondral or osteochondral lesions, and meniscal pathology.

CT can be a useful adjunct in patients with significant bony abnormalities who require further imaging when MRI is insufficient. CT can evaluate tunnel widening, bone tunnel integrity, and tunnel position. If significant tunnel widening is found, a staged bone grafting should be considered.

Results of Revision ACL Reconstruction

From a technical standpoint, results usually are not as good for revision ACL reconstructions as for primary procedures.[12] Because the goals of revision ACL surgery may differ from those of primary ACL reconstruction, a significant portion of preoperative counseling should be devoted to expectations.

Overall, results of revision ACL reconstruction show failure rates between 24% and 33%.[38-40] Two recent studies have reported lower failure rates of 3.4%[41] and 6%[42] following revision ACL reconstruction using both allograft and autograft tendons. The ability of patients to return to preinjury activities also is lower than expected with primary ACL reconstruction. As with primary ACL reconstruction, poorer outcomes can be expected in patients with significant articular or meniscus injuries.

Recent studies of combined ACL reconstruction and meniscal allograft transplantation have been reported. Sekiya and associates[43] reported on 28 patients, including nine with a combination ACL reconstruction and meniscal transplantation, with a follow-up of 2.8 years. Overall, 21 of the 28 patients achieved significant improvements after the combined surgery. No significant differences were found between primary and revision ACL reconstructions in subjective outcome, KT-1000 arthrometric testing (MEDmetric Corp, San Diego, CA), and functional testing. In addition, radiographic evaluation showed no significant joint space narrowing in the affected knee compared with the contralateral knee.

In an 8.5-year follow-up study, Graf and associates[44] reported the results of nine patients who underwent combined medial meniscal allograft transplantation and ACL reconstruction. In one patient, the meniscus was removed for presumed infection. International Knee Documentation Committee (IKDC) function tests showed six normal or near-normal scores and two abnormal scores. Six of the nine patients were still involved in recreational sports and pleased with their result. In selected patients with either chronic ACL deficiency or failed ACL reconstruction, restoration of meniscal function through allograft transplantation can provide satisfactory clinical results and may enhance joint stability and articular cartilage protection.

Preventing the Problem

ACL reconstruction is a technically demanding procedure that requires significant attention to detail. Preoperatively, ACL insufficiency and all associated problems must be recognized and addressed for a successful outcome. Any concomitant laxity must be treated to prevent excessive stress on the ACL graft. Any meniscal tear also should be repaired to prevent secondary osteoarthritis or future laxity. Because technical errors are the most common cause of ACL failure, careful attention to tunnel position, graft fixation, and graft tensioning is crucial. Finally, compliance with the rehabilitation protocol is necessary to protect the reconstructed graft in the early postoperative period.

Management and Outcome Summary

The patient in the case study required revision ACL reconstruction with patellar tendon-bone allograft and allograft meniscal transplantation using an endoscopic technique. Intraoperatively, the patient was confirmed to have medial meniscal deficiency with preserved articular surfaces and a chronic ACL deficiency (**Figure 8**). A double bone-plug technique was used for the allograft medial meniscus transplant, and the ACL reconstruction was performed with a BTB allograft using an all-endoscopic technique (**Figure 9**). Both the tibial and femoral interference screws were bypassed; therefore, screw removal was unnecessary. The graft was fixed with bioabsorbable interference screws on both the femoral and tibial sides.

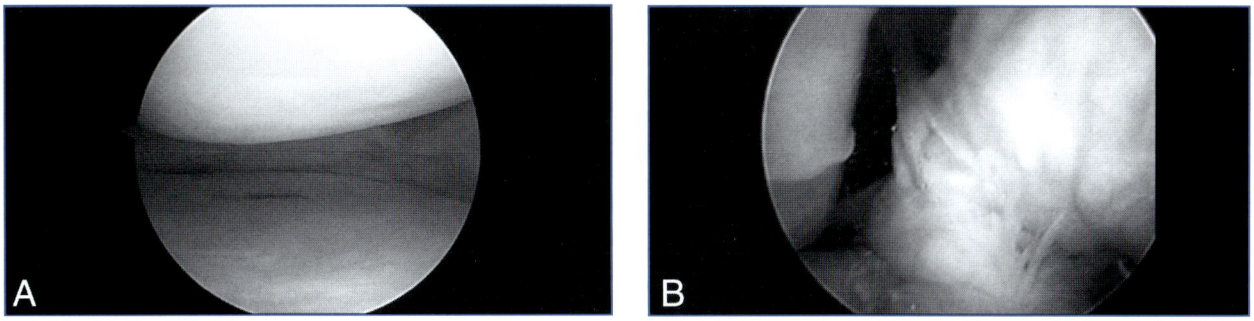

Figure 8 Intraoperative arthroscopic images showing a complete absence of the posterior horn of the medial meniscus with preservation of the articular cartilage surfaces **(A)** and absence of the ACL consistent with chronic ACL deficiency with graft failure **(B)**.

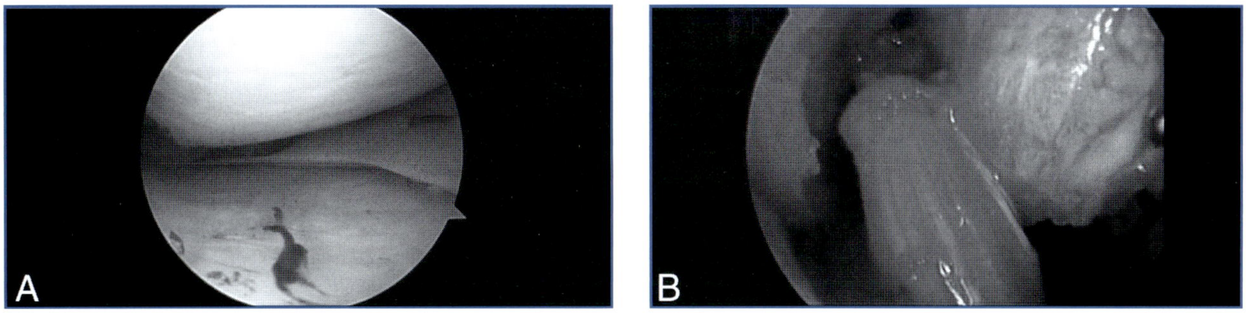

Figure 9 Intraoperative arthroscopic images showing the allograft medial meniscus transplant sewn in place with inside-out sutures **(A)** and the revision bone-patellar-bone allograft ACL reconstruction **(B)**.

Postoperatively, the patient was allowed partial weight bearing in full extension in a brace for the first 2 weeks and then advanced to full weight bearing as tolerated. In addition, his flexion was limited to 90° for the first 4 weeks. Four weeks postoperatively, he was allowed out of the brace, and flexion was advanced as tolerated. The patient achieved full knee ROM and leg strength by 3 months after surgery. At 6 months, he was allowed to return to full participation in sports without restrictions. Currently, he participates in recreational sports and no longer reports significant knee pain or instability.

Strategies to Minimize Common Complications

Because many ACL failures result from technical complications, careful attention to detail can prevent many revision situations. A complete preoperative evaluation for concomitant pathology, such as malalignment, meniscus or articular cartilage damage, and other ligamentous laxity, is crucial. In addition, the surgical principles during tunnel placement, graft tensioning, and graft fixation must be strictly followed to ensure the best outcome.

References

1. Azar FM: Revision anterior cruciate ligament reconstruction. *Instr Course Lect* 2002;51:335-342.
2. Harner CD, Giffin JR, Dunteman RC, Annunziata CC, Friedman MJ: Evaluation and treatment of recurrent instability after anterior cruciate ligament reconstruction. *Instr Course Lect* 2001;50:463-474.
3. Howell SM, Berns GS, Farley TE: Signal intensity measurements of unimpinged and impinged anterior cruciate ligament grafts. *Radiology* 1991;179:639-643.
4. Greis PE, Johnson DJ, Fu FH: Revision anterior cruciate ligament surgery: Cause of graft failure and technical considerations of revision surgery. *Clin Sports Med* 1993;12:839-852.
5. Jaureguito JW, Paulos LE: Why grafts fail? *Clin Orthop* 1996;325:25-41.
6. Getelman MH, Friedman MJ: Revision anterior cruciate ligament reconstruction surgery. *J Am Acad Orthop Surg* 1999;7:189-198.
7. O'Brien SJ, Warren RF, Pavlov H, Panariello R, Wickiewicz TL: Reconstruction of the chronically insufficient anterior cruciate ligament with the central third of the patellar ligament. *J Bone Joint Surg Am* 1991;73:278-286.
8. Maday MG, Harner CD, Fu FH: Revision ACL surgery: Evaluation and treatment, in Feagin JA Jr (ed): *Crucial Ligaments: Diagnosis and Treatment of Ligamentous Injuries About the Knee*. New York, NY, Churchill Livingstone, 1994, pp 711-723.
9. Burks RT, Leland R: Determination of graft tension before fixation in anterior cruciate ligament reconstruction. *Arthroscopy* 1988;4:260-266.
10. Gertel TH, Lew WD, Lewis JL Stewart NJ, Hunter RE: Effect of anterior cruciate ligament graft tensioning direction, magnitude, and flexion angle of knee biomechanics. *Am J Sports Med* 1993;21:572-581.
11. Johnson DL, Swanson TM, Irrgang JJ, Fu FH, Harner CD: Revision anterior cruciate ligament surgery: Experience from Pittsburgh. *Clin Orthop* 1996;325:100-109.
12. Uribe JW, Hechtman KS, Zvijac JE, Tjin-A-Tsoi EW: Revision anterior cruciate ligament surgery: Experience from Miami. *Clin Orthop* 1996;325:91-99.
13. Johnson DL, Harner CD, Fu FH: Revision anterior cruciate ligament surgery, in Harner CD, Fu FH, Vince KG (eds): *Knee Surgery*. Baltimore, MD, Williams & Wilkins, 1994, pp 877-895.
14. Howell SM, Clark JA, Farley TE: Serial magnetic resonance study assessing the effects of impingement on MR image of the patellar tendon graft. *Arthroscopy* 1992;8:350-358.
15. Ferrari JD, Bush-Joseph CA, Bach BR: Anterior cruciate ligament reconstruction using bone-patellar tendon-bone grafts: Autograft and allograft endoscopic techniques and two-incision autograft technique. *Oper Tech Sports Med* 1999;17:156-171.
16. Carson EW, Simonian PT, Wickiewicz TL, Warren RF: Revision anterior cruciate ligament reconstruction. *Instr Course Lect* 1998;47:361-368.
17. Morgan CD, Kalman VR, Grawl DM: Definitive anatomic landmarks for tibial tunnel positioning for ACL reconstruction. *Arthroscopy* 1995;11:275-288.
18. Melby A III, Noble JS, Askew MJ, Boom AA, Hurst FW: The effects of graft tensioning on the laxity and kinematics of the anterior cruciate ligament reconstructed knee. *Arthroscopy* 1991;7:257-266.
19. Asahina S, Muneta T, Ishibashi T, Yamamoto H: Effects of knee flexion angle at graft fixation on the outcome of anterior cruciate ligament reconstruction. *Arthroscopy* 1996;12:70-75.
20. Bylski-Austrow DI, Grood ES, Hefzy MS, Holden JP, Butler DL: Anterior cruciate ligament replacements: A mechanical study of femoral attachment location, flexion angle at tensioning, and initial tension. *J Orthop Res* 1990;8:522-531.
21. Yoshiya S, Andrish JY, Manley MT, Bauer TW: Graft tension in anterior cruciate ligament reconstruction: An in vivo study in dogs. *Am J Sports Med* 1987;15:464-470.
22. Schabus R, Fuchs M, Kwasny O: The effect of ACL-graft preload on the static pressure distribution in the knee-joint. *Orthop Trans* 1989;13:431-432.
23. Tredinnick TJ, Friedman MJ: Revision anterior cruciate ligament reconstruction: Technical considerations. *Am J Knee Surg* 2001;14:193-200.
24. Johnson DL, Miller MD, Fu FH: The arthroscopic "impingement test" during anterior cruciate ligament reconstruction. *Arthroscopy* 1993;9:714-717.
25. Butler DL: Evaluation of fixation methods in cruciate ligament replacements. *Instr Course Lect* 1987;36:173-178.
26. Kurosaka M, Yoshiya S, Andrish JT: A biomechanical comparison of different surgical techniques of graft fixation in anterior cruciate ligament reconstruction. *Am J Sports Med* 1987;12:225-229.

27. Wetzler MJ, et al: Revision anterior cruciate ligament surgery: Etiology of failures. *Oper Tech Sports Med* 1998;6:64-70.

28. Drez DJ Jr, DeLee J, Holden JP, Arnoczky S, Noyes FR, Roberts TS: Anterior cruciate ligament reconstruction using bone-patellar tendon-bone allografts: A biological and biomechanical evaluation in goats. *Am J Sports Med* 1991;19:256-263.

29. Rodeo SA, Arnoczky SP, Torzilli PA, Hidake C, Warren RF: Tendon-healing in a bone tunnel: A biomechanical and histological study in the dog. *J Bone Joint Surg Am* 1993;75:1795-1803.

30. Noyes FR, Barber-Westin SD, Roberts CS: Use of allografts after failed treatment of rupture of the anterior cruciate ligament. *J Bone Joint Surg Am* 1994;76:1019-1031.

31. Arnoczky SP: Biology of ACL reconstructions: What happens to the graft. *Instr Course Lect* 1996;45:229-233.

32. Yoshiya S, Nagano M, Kurosaka M, Muratsu H, Mizuno K: Graft healing in the bone tunnel in anterior cruciate ligament reconstruction. *Clin Orthop* 2000;376: 278-286.

33. Cosgarea AJ, DeHaven KE, Lovelock JE: The surgical treatment of arthrofibrosis of the knee. *Am J Sports Med* 1994;22:184-191.

34. Williams RJ III, Laurencin CT, Warren RF, Speciale AC, Brause BD, O'Brien S: Septic arthritis after anterior crucicate ligament reconstruction: Diagnosis and management. *Am J Sports Med* 1997;25:261-267.

35. DeHaven KE, Cosgarea AJ, Sebastianelli WJ: Arthrofibrosis of the knee following ligament surgery. *Instr Course Lect* 2003;52:369-381.

36. Noyes FR, Barber-Westin SD: Revision anterior cruciate surgery with use of bone-patellar tendon-bone autogenous grafts. *J Bone Joint Surg Am* 2001;83:1131-1143.

37. Noyes FR, Barber-Westin SD, Hewett TE: High tibial osteotomy and ligament reconstruction for varus angulated anterior cruciate ligament-deficient knees. *Am J Sports Med* 2000;28:282-296.

38. Noyes FR, Barber-Westin SD, Roberts CS: Use of allografts after failed treatment of rupture of the anterior cruciate ligament. *J Bone Joint Surg Am* 1994;76:1019-1031.

39. Noyes FR, Barber-Westin SD: Revision anterior cruciate surgery with use of bone-patellar tendon-bone autogenous grafts. *J Bone Joint Surg Am* 2001;83:1131-1143.

40. Fox JA, Pierce M, Bojchuk J, Hayden J, Bush-Joseph CA, Bach BR: Revision anterior cruciate ligament reconstruction with nonirradiated fresh-frozen patellar tendon allograft. *Arthroscopy* 2004;20:787-794.

41. Grossman MG, ElAttrache NS, Shields CL, Glousman RE: Revision anterior cruciate ligament reconstruction: Three- to nine-year follow-up. *Arthroscopy* 2005;21:418-423.

42. O'Neill DB: Revision arthroscopically assisted anterior cruciate ligament reconstruction with previously unharvested ipsilateral autografts. *Am J Sports Med* 2005;32:1833-1841.

43. Sekiya J, Giffin JR, Irrgang JJ, Fu FH, Harner CD: Clinical outcomes after combined meniscal allograft transplantation and anterior cruciate ligament reconstruction. *Am J Sports Med* 2003;31: 896-906.

44. Graf KW Jr, Sekiya JK, Wojtys EM: Long-term results after combined medial meniscal allograft transplantation and anterior cruciate ligament reconstruction: Minimum 8.5-year follow-up study. *Arthroscopy* 2004;20:129-140.

Chapter 7

Technical Aspects of Revision ACL Reconstruction

Ronald Edward Glenn, Jr, MD
Bernard R. Bach, Jr, MD

Case Presentation

History

A 15-year-old female soccer player heard a pop in her right knee as she was struck by another player while her right foot was planted on the field. She was unable to bear weight on the leg and noted immediate swelling of the knee. Physical examination revealed an obvious effusion, a grade IIB Lachman test, and diffuse medial knee tenderness. MRI showed a complete rupture of the anterior cruciate ligament (ACL) and a medial collateral ligament sprain with an intact posterior cruciate ligament (PCL) and intact menisci.

The patient subsequently underwent endoscopic ACL reconstruction by another surgeon, who used a fresh frozen, irradiated bone-patellar tendon-bone allograft.

Current Problem and Treatment

The patient initially did well after surgery but reported atraumatic knee instability with deceleration activities and transient swelling of the knee after cutting or pivoting. Physical examination revealed 0° to 140° of knee flexion, a grade I Lachman test, a grade II anterior drawer test, and a grade I pivot-shift test. KT-1000 arthrometer (MEDmetric Corporation, San Diego, CA) testing revealed a side-to-side difference of 2, 4, and 8 mm, respectively, of anterior translation at 15 lb, 20 lb, and maximum manual testing. Radiographs of the knee demonstrated a posteriorly oriented tibial tunnel and a vertically oriented femoral tunnel (**Figure 1**). A repeat MRI scan revealed an intact ACL with vertical orientation and no other concomitant intra-articular pathology.

The patient was diagnosed with a failed ACL reconstruction resulting from improper tunnel placement. Treatment at this time was to consist of examination under anesthesia and subsequent revision ACL reconstruction with a fresh frozen, nonirradiated bone-patellar tendon-bone allograft, if the examination was consistent with the preoperative diagnosis.

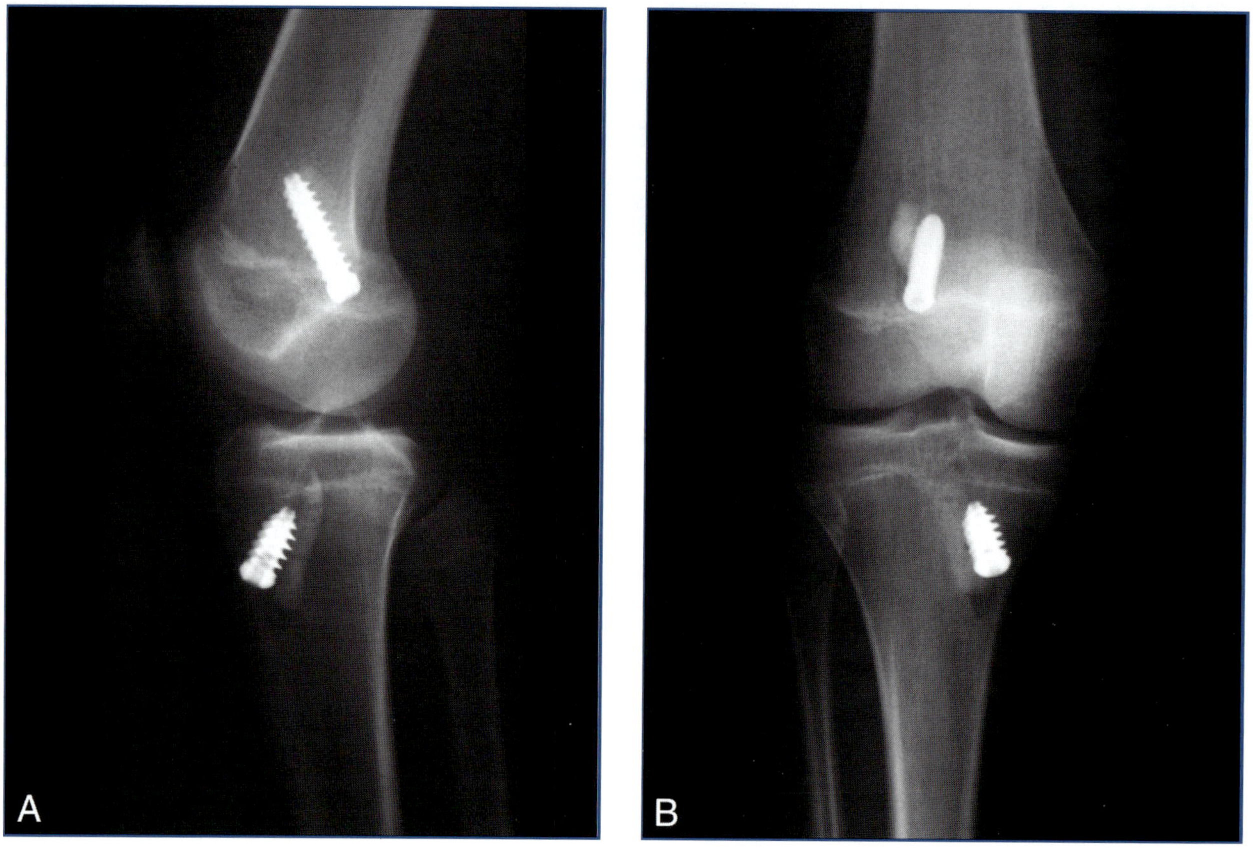

Figure 1 AP view of the right knee **(A)** shows a vertically oriented graft on the femur, and the lateral view **(B)** shows that the orientation of the tibial bone plug is too posterior. These observations are common in endoscopic ACL failure. Note that the femoral placement of the bone plug appears appropriate on the lateral radiograph.

Discussion

Recognizing the Problem

ACL reconstruction is one of the most commonly performed surgeries in orthopaedics; however, the number of failures reported is increasing as more reconstructions are being performed.[1-5] At short- and intermediate-term follow-up, failure rates are reported to range from 10% to 15%.[6-8] For this discussion, failure is defined as a clinically unstable and symptomatic knee secondary to ACL incompetence characterized by an abnormal Lachman test, a positive pivot-shift test, and abnormal side-to-side differences on KT-1000 arthrometer testing.

Assessment of a possible failed ACL reconstruction must begin with identifying the primary cause of failure. A thorough history and physical examination rule out associated knee or concomitant hip or low back pathology, and radiographs often reveal the cause of graft failure. Whether the femoral and tibial tunnels are in an anatomic position, or whether they are expanded should be investigated. Nonanatomic tunnels that do not overlap the anatomic position usually are easily revised, whereas nonanatomic overlapping tunnels may require bone grafting[9] (**Figure 2**). If radiographs show tunnel expansion (**Figure 3**), CT can be obtained to better define the amount of bone loss. Because tunnel expansion occurs more commonly with the use of hamstrings graft, Achilles tendon allograft, and synthetic graft (Gore-Tex [Gore Creative Technologies Worldwide, Newark, DE] or ligament augmentation device), CT should be considered, even if bone loss is not apparent on plain radiographs.[10]

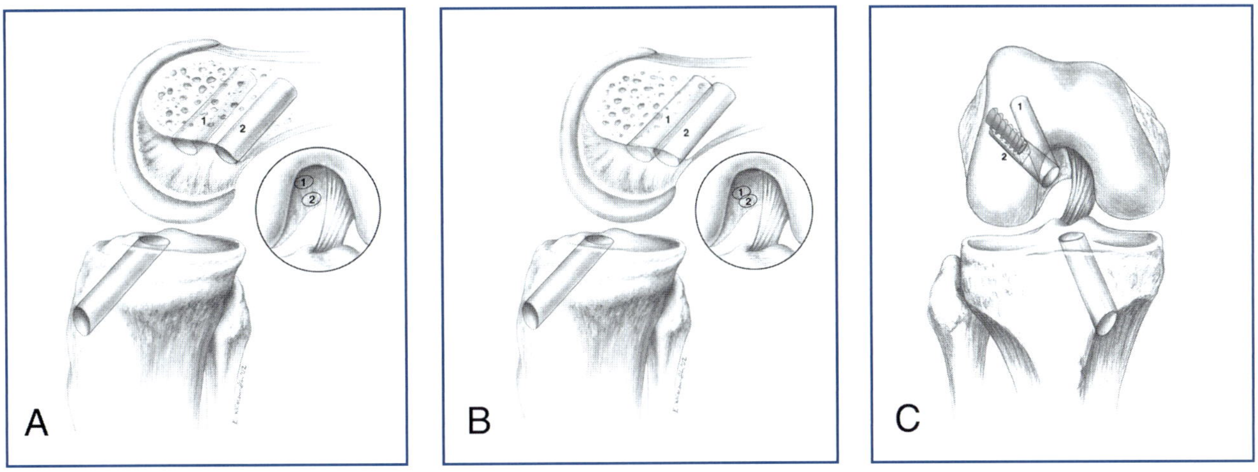

Figure 2 **A,** Nonoverlapping, nonanatomic femoral tunnels. Tunnel 1 represents an anterior malposition, and tunnel 2 shows that a revision could be performed without violation of tunnel 1. **B,** Overlapping tunnels. In this figure, tunnel 1 represents the index femoral tunnel, and tunnel 2 shows the proper location for the revision femoral tunnel. In this situation, the tunnels are likely to overlap, which may require primary or staged bone grafting, or stacking the graft fixation with an additional screw. **C,** AP view of the right knee shows how a different orientation of the tunnel could result in a similar intra-articular placement of the graft. The revision tunnel (2) could be created with an outside-in approach, or an inside-out (endoscopic) approach if an accessory inferomedial portal is used and the knee is hyperflexed. (Reproduced from Bach BR Jr, Fox JA, Mazzocca AD: Revision ACL reconstruction. *Orthopaedic Knowledge Online*. Rosemont, Illinois, American Academy of Orthopaedic Surgeons, 2002.)

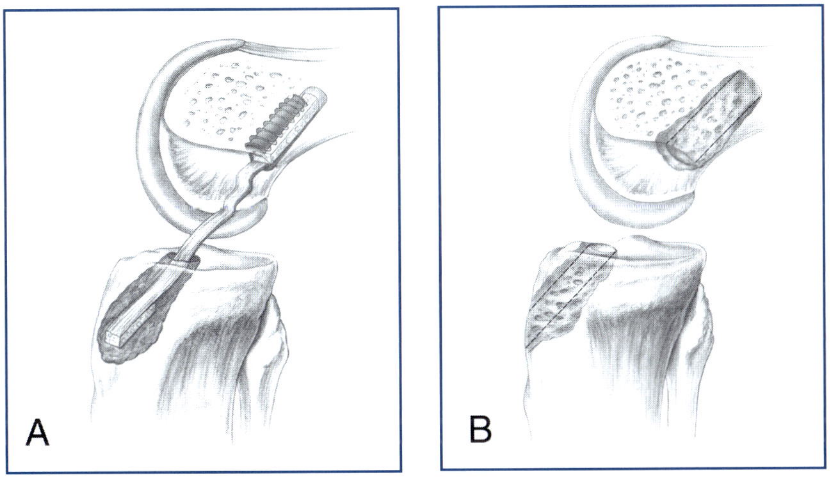

Figure 3 This lateral view of the knee illustrates tibial tunnel expansion **(A)** and staged bone grafting of expanded tibial and femoral tunnels **(B)**. (Reproduced from Bach BR Jr, Fox JA, Mazzocca AD: Revision ACL reconstruction. *Orthopaedic Knowledge Online.* Rosemont, Illinois, American Academy of Orthopaedic Surgeons, 2002.)

Management of the Problem

Preoperative Planning

Once the decision has been made to proceed with revision ACL reconstruction, thorough preoperative planning is essential. A review of the index procedure is important to identify any associated intra-articular pathology and how it was addressed at that time. It also may describe any difficulties encountered during the initial ACL reconstruction. Evaluating the current tunnel position is important to determine if the preexisting hardware needs to be removed.

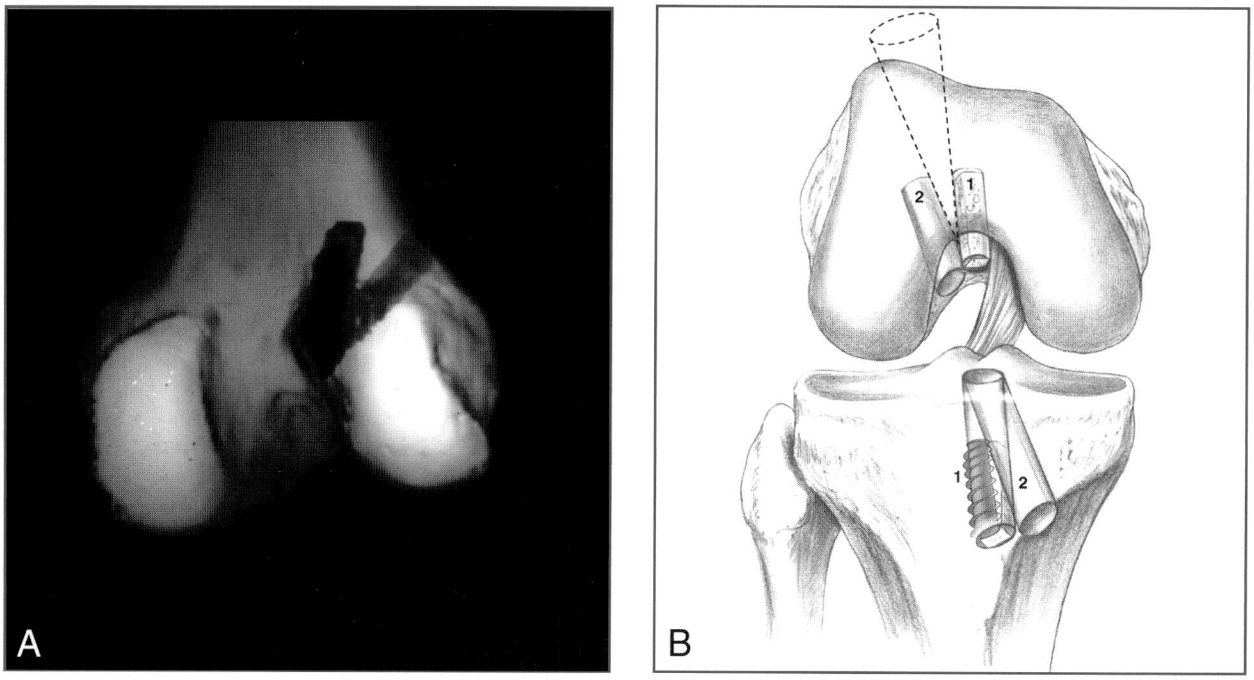

Figure 4 The divergent tunnel or "funnel" concept in which the correct intra-articular position may be achieved with a different starting orientation. **A,** CT scan shows both endoscopic and outside-in approaches were used to create respective tunnels with the same intra-articular location. (Reproduced with permission from Dworsky B, Jewell BF, Bach BR Jr: Interference screw divergence in endoscopic anterior cruciate ligament reconstruction. *Arthroscopy* 1996;12:45-49.) **B,** The initial tunnels (1) were oriented too much in the sagittal plane, resulting in a vertically oriented femoral tunnel. Tunnel 2 was created at revision to illustrate the divergent tunnel concept. (Reproduced from Bach BR Jr, Fox JA, Mazzocca AD: Revision ACL reconstruction. *Orthopaedic Knowledge Online.* Rosemont, Illinois, American Academy of Orthopaedic Surgeons, 2002.)

Radiographs of the tunnels will indicate whether bone graft is needed to fill any defects in the femur or tibia as a result of tunnel expansion. In some instances, a staged reconstruction may be required to address the bony deficit before proceeding with ligament reconstruction.

The divergent tunnel or "funnel" concept should be mentioned here.[9,10] The anatomic intra-articular femoral and tibial entry points can be approached from several different extra-articular orientations. If the angle or position selected for drilling differs from that used for the index procedure, the surgeon can select the proper site for tunnel placement and then diverge or "funnel" away from the original tunnel with minimal overlap. Understanding the funnel concept is important when deciding if preexisting hardware needs to be removed or if it can be bypassed; it also can help determine if bone grafting is needed to aid in ligament fixation. An understanding of this concept also may help the surgeon determine whether revision ACL reconstruction should be performed endoscopically or with a two-incision technique. For example, although the same femoral intra-articular entry point can be obtained using either an endoscopic or a two-incision technique, the directions of the extra-articular femoral tunnel are quite different. When the tibial tunnel is placed in an excessive sagittal orientation, a more medial tibial tunnel may be created using the concept of diverging tunnels, which provides an intact tube of bone in the tibia for more secure fixation (**Figure 4**).

In general, two-incision ACL reconstructions and most endoscopic ACL reconstructions can be revised endoscopically. A two-incision technique may be needed for a patient with a failed endoscopic ACL reconstruction secondary to posterior wall blowout or overlapping tunnels because both may affect graft fixation.[9] The two-incision technique provides diverging tunnels for an intact tube of bone on the femoral side and ultimately adequate graft fixation.

Graft Selection

Graft selection is another important preoperative consideration. A variety of graft options, including autografts and allografts, is available. The latter may be irradiated or nonirradiated.[11,12] Graft choices include patellar tendon, hamstrings tendon, quadriceps tendon, tibialis anterior tendon, and Achilles tendon. If the index procedure was a hamstrings reconstruction, use of an ipsilateral patellar tendon autograft could be considered. In general, we believe that a hamstrings graft is not an ideal choice for revision ACL reconstruction because the tunnels are frequently expanded, and secure graft fixation (such as that obtained with bone plugs and interference screws) cannot be obtained consistently. We prefer a nonirradiated patellar tendon allograft. A patellar tendon allograft allows for customization of both graft size and bone plug size, it provides additional bone graft to fill prior tunnel defects, it allows for interference screw fixation on both sides of the joint, and it is associated with low morbidity.[4] If allograft tissue is used, its associated risks and benefits should be discussed with the patient, and informed consent should be obtained. In addition, when requesting allograft tissue, the patient's height and an estimate of graft length are needed to prevent a significant graft-host mismatch. A patellar tendon autograft should not be reharvested for revision ACL reconstruction if one was used in the index procedure because the tissue has been shown to be suboptimal.[13]

Technique

Decisions regarding the type of reconstruction (endoscopic versus two-incision), graft type, hardware removal, and bone graft requirements should be made preoperatively. If allograft tissue is chosen, graft availability should be confirmed before surgery. If hardware removal is a possibility, a variety of screwdrivers should be available given the different types of screw head recesses.[14] Instrumentation also should be readily available to facilitate removal of screws that may be stripped. A thorough examination of the knee with the patient under anesthesia is indicated to rule out any associated pathology. In addition, the patient should be positioned so that the surgeon can flex the knee to at least 110° to ensure proper femoral tunnel placement during surgery.

Next, standard anteromedial and anterolateral portals are established, and a complete diagnostic arthroscopy is performed. Associated meniscal and chondral pathology should be addressed at the time of surgery. Once ACL incompetence has been confirmed arthroscopically, the residual ACL should be completely débrided to visualize the tibial footprint, the lateral wall of the intercondylar notch, and the over-the-top position on the distal femur. Use of the arthroscopic scissors, shaver, osteotome, and electrocautery will help facilitate the débridement. A notchplasty should be performed to prevent graft impingement laterally in the intercondylar notch, as well as superiorly on the roof of the intercondylar notch.

Tibial Tunnel

Attention should then be turned to the tibial tunnel. The tibial guide is typically set at 50° to 55° so that the entry point of the guide pin is at least 2 to 2.5 cm below the joint line. The intra-articular portion of the tibial guide should be positioned so that the guide wire enters the joint in the intercondylar notch at the level of the posterior edge of the anterior horn of the lateral meniscus and approximately 7 mm anterior to the origin of the PCL. To prevent a tibial tunnel that is too vertical in the sagittal plane, an accessory inferomedial portal or transpatellar portal may be required to place the tibial guide in a proper position (**Figure 5**, *A*). Once the intra-articular portion of the tibial guide has been placed in the appropriate position, the extra-articular portion should be positioned so that a long tibial tunnel can be created. An entrance site beginning midway between the tibial tubercle and the posteromedial corner of the tibia will produce appropriate tibial tunnel orientation in the coronal plane.[10] The guide pin is advanced through the tibia into the knee joint, and the position of the pin is confirmed arthroscopically (**Figure 5**, *B*). An incision is then made to

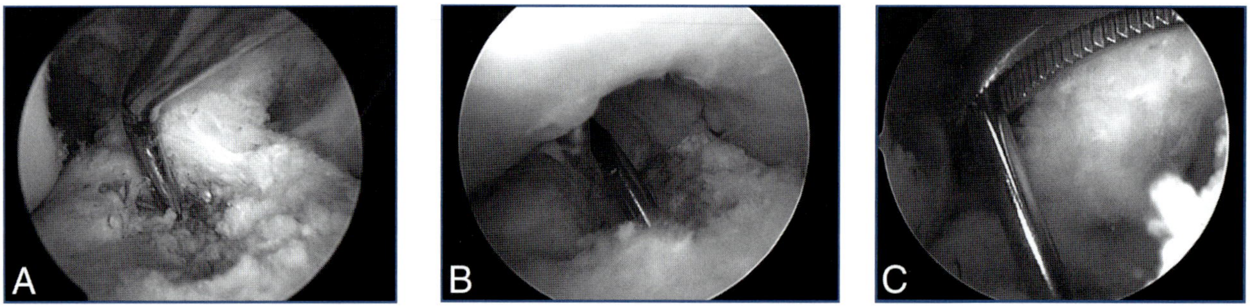

Figure 5 **A,** The tibial aimer usually is introduced through an accessory inferomedial portal. Reference points for pin placement include the posterior edge of the anterior horn of the lateral meniscus and the PCL. **B,** Once the pin is drilled, its position is checked by extending the knee to ensure that the pin is posterior to the intercondylar apex in extension. **C,** The pin is stabilized with a Kocher clamp before reaming if it has been drilled through a significant portion of the previous tibial tunnel.

expose the medial tibial metaphyseal region. At this point a decision is made regarding hardware removal. If the prior tibial tunnel can be easily bypassed, the hardware is left in place. If the hardware blocks the path of the new tibial tunnel, it must be removed. Fluoroscopy may be required to identify the previous hardware if it is not readily visible. If the tunnels overlap and the bony bridge between the new and old tunnels is not sufficient, the old screw may be temporarily removed and replaced at the time of graft fixation to the tibia, essentially stacking the old and new interference screws. Alternatively, the old tibial tunnel may be bone grafted and a single interference screw used. Ideally, a separate tibial tunnel with an adequate bony bridge is created so that bone grafting is not necessary, and a single interference screw can be used for tibial fixation.

As the tibial guide pin is advanced into the knee joint, it often will encounter the prior tibial tunnel as it traverses the tibia. The guide pin should be stabilized in the joint with a Kocher clamp or advanced into the femur to prevent any micromotion of the pin during tibial reaming (**Figure** 5, C). The new tibial tunnel is created using an 11-mm cannulated reamer, which is slowly advanced into the knee joint under arthroscopic visualization to ensure proper tunnel placement. The intra-articular portion of the tibial tunnel is débrided with an arthroscopic shaver passed retrograde into the tibial tunnel or smoothed with a rasp to prevent abrasion of the graft by the posterior and posterolateral portions of the tibial tunnel. The tunnel is then inspected with the arthroscope. If the newly formed tibial tunnel is in continuity with the previous tunnel, separate bone graft or a larger tibial bone plug is required to fill the defect and allow for an interference fit with tibial fixation.

Femoral Tunnel

Attention is next directed to creation of the femoral tunnel. As with the tibial tunnel, a decision about hardware removal must be made. If the femoral tunnel is in the appropriate location, it may be reused (**Figure 6**). If only the intra-articular entry point is in the appropriate location, the divergent tunnel concept is used. If the femoral tunnel is in a nonanatomic position, the hardware may be bypassed and an entirely new femoral tunnel created. If hardware removal is needed, any bone around the periphery of the screw must be removed to facilitate screw removal and prevent stripping. A flexible wire is then placed into the cannulated screw through the anteromedial or accessory inferomedial portal with the knee in flexion, and the screwdriver is directed over the wire into the screw head for removal. If the screw is vertically oriented, the hardware may be bypassed by slightly advancing the screw.

Any remaining soft tissue along the lateral wall of the intercondylar notch is removed, and the over-the-top position (1 o'clock position in the left knee; 11 o'clock position in the right knee) is confirmed by palpation with an arthroscopic probe. With the inflow turned off and the knee dry, a 7-mm femoral

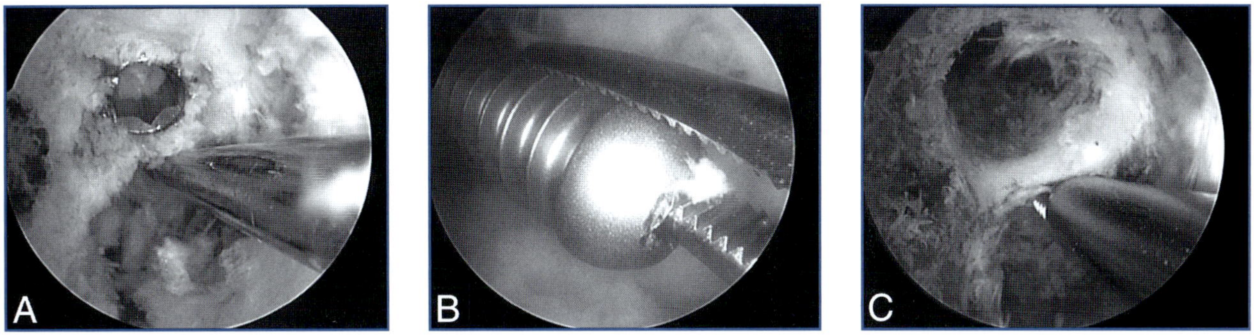

Figure 6 **A,** Arthroscopic image obtained during revision ACL reconstruction shows a well-placed femoral tunnel. This requires screw removal so that the tunnel can be used again. **B,** The screw is removed, and the tunnel is redrilled **(C)**.

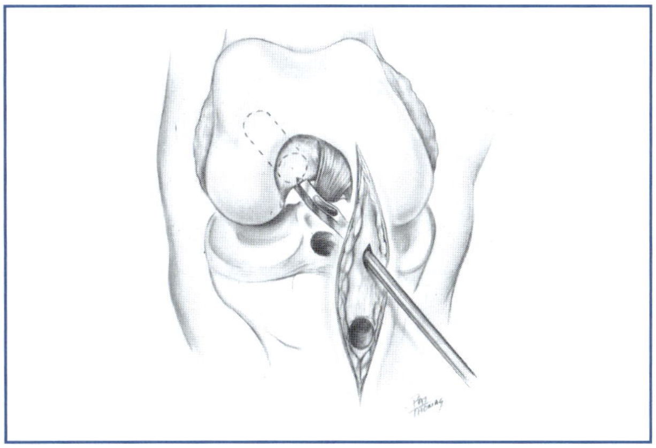

Figure 7 Use of an accessory inferomedial portal to create the femoral tunnel. Note that if this modified approach is used, the knee must be flexed to 110° to decrease the likelihood of drilling out the posterior cortex. (Reproduced from Bach BR Jr, Fox JA, Mazzocca AD: Revision ACL reconstruction. *Orthopaedic Knowledge Online*. Rosemont, Illinois, American Academy of Orthopaedic Surgeons, 2002.)

offset guide is placed retrograde through the tibial tunnel to the corresponding over-the-top position on the femur with the knee flexed 80°. If the tibial tunnel forces the femoral offset guide into an unacceptable vertical position on the femur, the accessory inferomedial portal may be used with the knee in 110° of hyperflexion to obtain the correct femoral tunnel starting position[15] (**Figure** 7).

During drilling, the PCL is protected with an arthroscopic probe. A 3/32-inch Steinmann pin is provisionally drilled into the femur approximately 3 to 4 cm, a 10-mm cannulated reamer is then placed over the guide pin, and the femoral tunnel is reamed to a depth of 5 to 7 mm to create an endoscopic footprint. The reamer is then removed, and the footprint is visualized arthroscopically to confirm an intact posterior wall. When using a 7-mm offset guide, a 10-mm reamer should provide 2 mm of intact posterior wall. Once the posterior wall is confirmed to be intact, the reamer is advanced retrograde into the femur approximately 35 mm. If the previous and current femoral tunnels are overlapping, bone graft can be used to fill the defect left by the previous tunnel. The reamer and guide pin are removed, and the arthroscope is placed retrograde up the tibial tunnel or through the accessory inferomedial portal into the newly created femoral tunnel. The femoral tunnel is then inspected to ensure an intact posterior wall along the entire course of the tunnel. Any remaining soft tissue from the prior femoral tunnel should be removed if the tunnels overlap.

In the case of a femoral tunnel with a posterior wall blowout, the two-incision technique should be considered to create a new femoral tunnel with an intact bony tube to allow for secure graft fixation (**Figure** 8). For the two-incision technique, a laterally based incision is made beginning at the proximal pole of the patella and extending proximally 1.5 inches (**Figure** 9). The skin and subcutaneous tissues are divided, exposing the iliotibial band. A 2-inch longitudinal incision is made in the midsubstance of the iliotibial band, and the vastus lateralis muscle is bluntly elevated anteriorly with a finger. A Z-knee retractor is then placed to retract the vastus lateralis

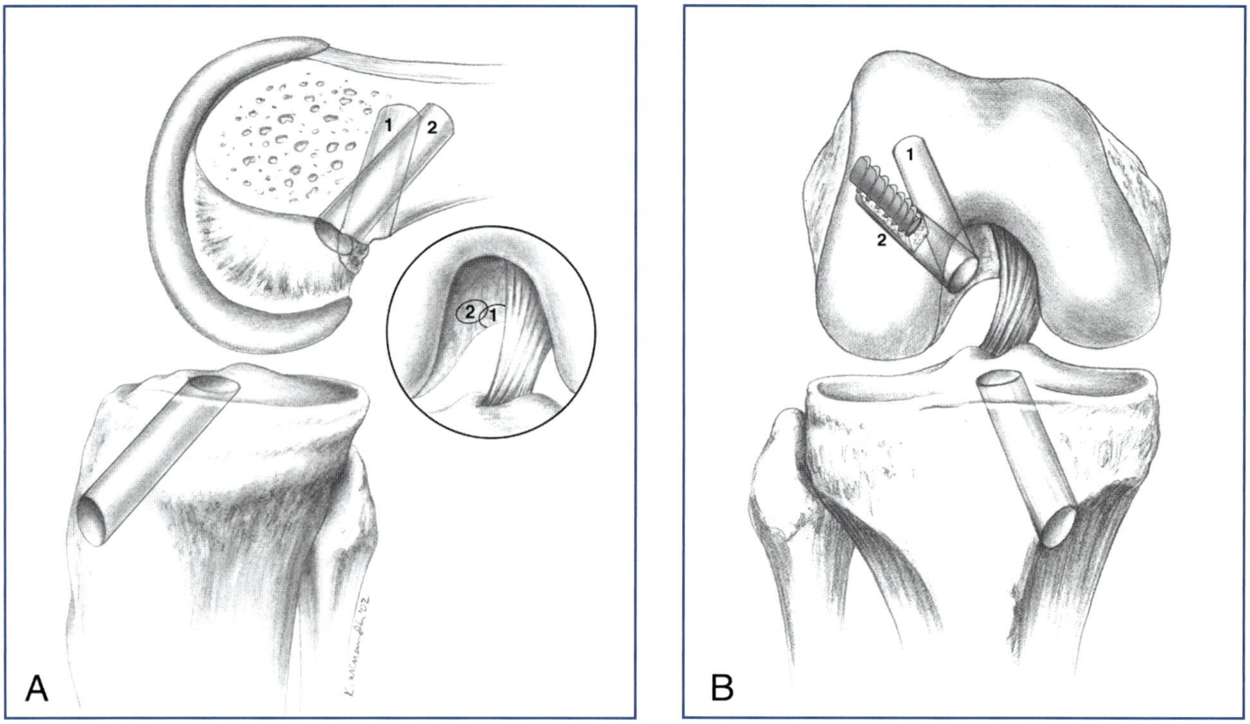

Figure 8 **A,** The creation of tunnel 1 resulted in violation of the posterior cortex. The amount of violation or "blowout" can vary both in depth and circumference. These variables may impact the decision to convert to a two-incision approach. **B,** Use of a two-incision femoral tunnel provides adequate femoral fixation when a posterior wall blowout occurs.

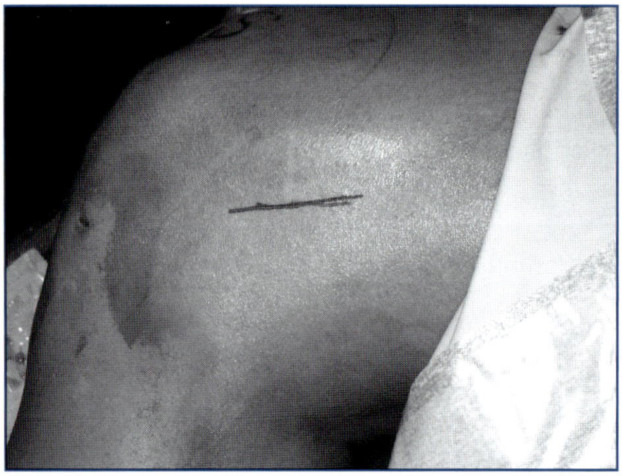

Figure 9 A lateral incision is made for a two-incision approach.

anteriorly. The periosteum is longitudinally divided with electrocautery, and subperiosteal dissection is continued with a Cobb elevator so that the over-the-top position can be palpated. A J-shaped femoral guide passer is then inserted through the anterolateral portal into the intercondylar notch and around the over-the-top position such that the instrument pops through the joint capsule anterior to the lateral intermuscular septum. The rear-entry femoral guide is attached to the guide passer and is directed into the intercondylar notch by removing the guide passer from the knee through the anterolateral arthroscopic portal in the opposite direction to that in which it was inserted. The rear-entry guide is then placed in the over-the-top position, and the provisional femoral guide pin is inserted into the distal femur under arthroscopic visualization. A 10-mm cannulated reamer is used to drill the femoral tunnel.[9]

Graft Preparation

Once the tibial and femoral tunnels have been created, the graft is prepared. If a patellar tendon allograft is used, any excess fat is removed from the tendon. The total length of the graft is generally 95 to 105 mm. The bone plugs should measure around 25 mm in length.[4] If the tunnels are overlapping or expanded, the bone plugs can be contoured in a normal fashion to slide easily through a 10-mm sizing tube, and the remaining allograft bone can be used as graft material. Bone grafting of the femoral tunnel should be performed through a clear cannula, and the graft should be packed tightly into the tunnel to create a firm osseous tunnel. A second option is to fashion cortical allograft matchsticks to place into the defect[9] (**Figure 10**, *A*). A third option with patellar tendon allograft is to leave the bone plugs large to fill the tunnel defects. Alternatively, screws may be stacked to enhance fixation of the bone plug when overlapping or expanded tunnels are encountered (**Figure 10**, *B*).

With the knee flexed approximately 80°, an instrument is used to advance the femoral bone plug through the tibial tunnel into the joint. A hemostat is then placed through the medial portal, and the femoral bone plug is grasped at the junction of the proximal and middle thirds and advanced into the femoral tunnel with the graft oriented so that the cortical side of the bone plug is facing posteriorly and the cancellous side is facing anteriorly. Alternatively, the graft can be advanced using a "pull-through" technique by placing a Beath pin through both tunnels and advancing the graft using traction sutures. The graft is not completely seated so that the plug may act as a skid for the flexible guide wire that is inserted through the accessory inferomedial portal into the femoral tunnel anterior to the femoral plug. The knee is then hyperflexed to 100° to 110°, and the wire is advanced until it bottoms out at the end of the femoral tunnel. Completely advancing the pin ensures parallel placement of the femoral interference screw. The knee is then brought back down to 80° of flexion, and the femoral plug is advanced until it sits flush in the notch. A mark placed at the bone-tendon interface during graft preparation will aid in determining complete seating of the bone plug.

At this time, graft length is assessed for graft-patient mismatch. If no mismatch is noted, the femoral bone plug is fixed with a 7- × 25-mm metal cannulated interference screw (**Figure 11**). If the bone is osteopenic, a 9- × 25-mm screw can be used. Fixation should be performed with the knee in 110° of hyperflexion to prevent nonparallel placement of the interference screw and potential screw breakout through the posterior femur.[4] If a construct mismatch is noted, several options can remedy the situation, including advancement of the femoral bone plug prior to fixation, graft rotation up to 540° after femoral fixation (which can effectively shorten the graft length by 6 to 8 mm), or use of a free bone block technique.[9]

After the femoral plug has been secured, the fixation is tested by placing manual tension distally on the graft. The graft is then cycled multiple times with tension held on the graft throughout the knee range of motion. Isometry should be assessed at this time. If placed properly, the graft should be pulled into the tibial tunnel approximately 1 to 2 mm as the knee moves through the terminal 20° of extension.

Tibial fixation is now performed. The graft should be rotated 180° and oriented so that the cancellous side of the bone plug is facing posteriorly, and the cortical side of the bone plug is facing anteriorly. While holding tension on the tibial plug to prevent twisting, a 9- × 20-mm or 9- × 25-mm tibial interference screw is placed anterior to the bone plug with the knee in full extension. Anterior screw placement is less likely to abrade the tendinous portion of the graft if the screw extends past the tibial bone plug.[4] If the tibial bone plug is recessed within the tibial tunnel during fixation of the femoral tunnel, a longer tibial interference screw should be used rather than burying a shorter screw. Expanded tunnels can be addressed as previously mentioned with bone graft, a larger bone plug, or stacking interference screws. If adequate tibial fixation is still a concern, a screw-and-post construct or a Hewson Ligament Button (Richards, Memphis, TN) may be used.[9]

Once the ligament reconstruction is secured on the femoral and tibial sides, the knee is cycled multiple times, and fixation is assessed. Lachman, anterior drawer, and pivot-shift tests are performed before wound closure. The graft is then inspected visually

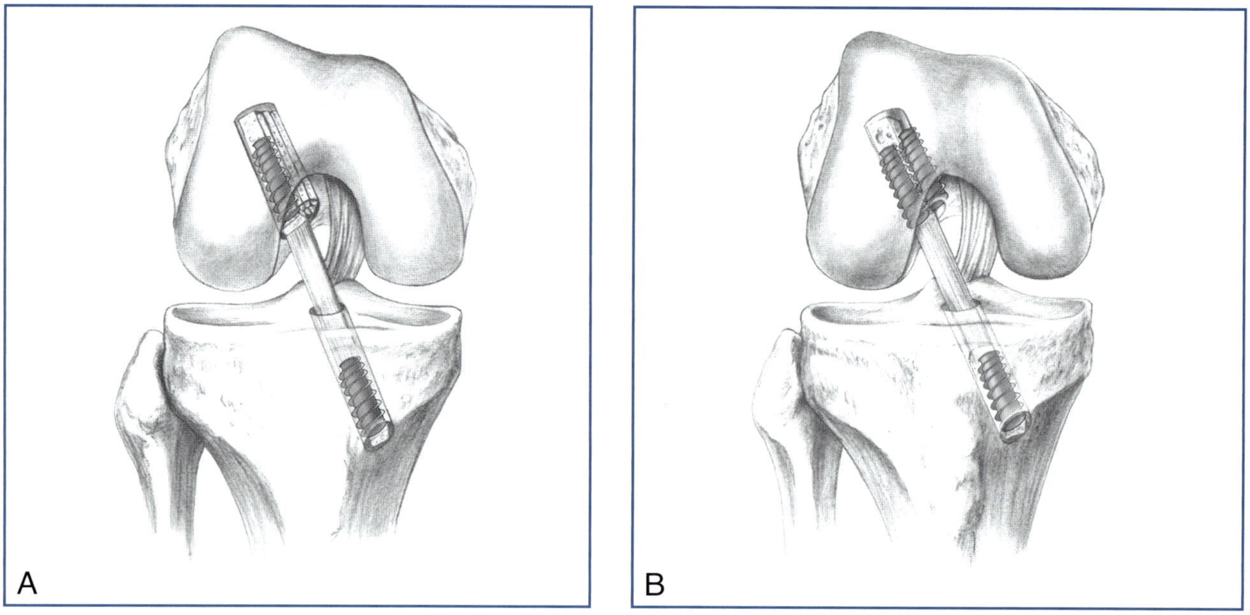

Figure 10 **A,** Bone grafting performed with allograft "matchsticks" for an enlarged femoral tunnel. **B,** Another approach for patients with slightly enlarged femoral tunnels or with overlapping tunnels is the addition of another or "stacked" interference screws. (Reproduced from Bach BR Jr, Fox JA, Mazzocca AD: Revision ACL reconstruction. *Orthopaedic Knowledge Online.* Rosemont, Illinois, American Academy of Orthopaedic Surgeons, 2002.)

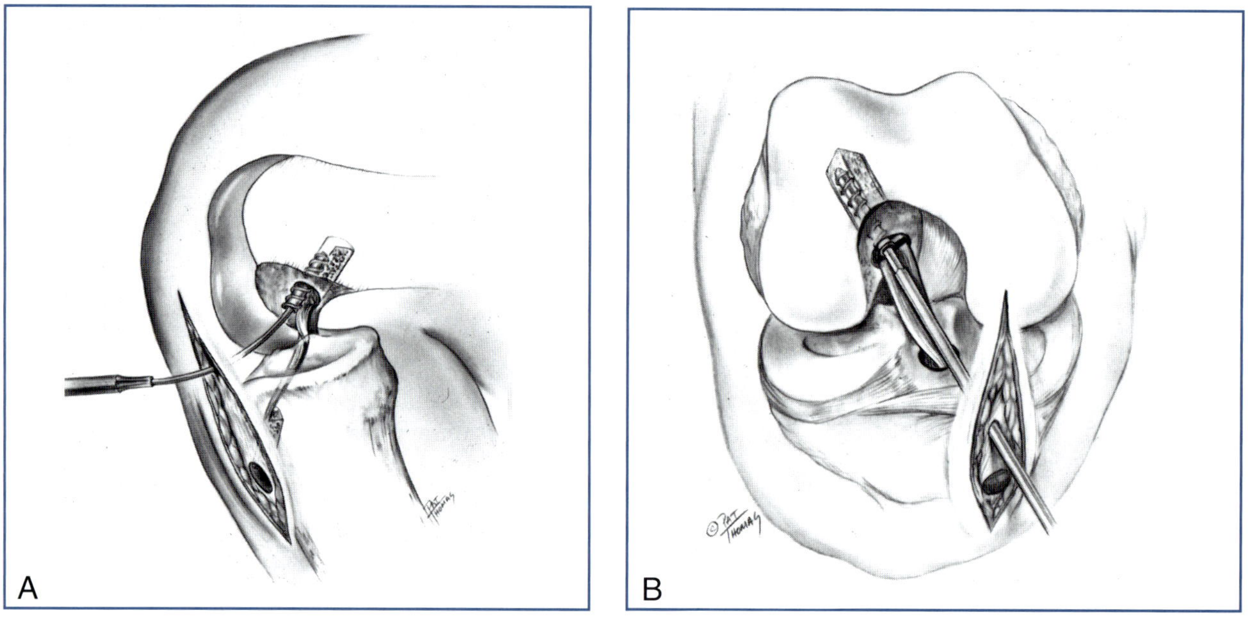

Figure 11 **A,** A flexible wire is inserted through an accessory inferomedial portal or the original inferomedial portal and placed in the interval between the femoral socket and the femoral bone plug. The knee is then flexed, and the pin is advanced prior to insertion of the interference screw. **B,** Placement of the interference screw. (Reproduced with permission from Hardin GT, Bach BR Jr, Bush-Joseph, Farr J: Endoscopic single incision ACL reconstruction using patellar tendon autograft-surgical technique. *Am J Knee Surg* 1992;5:144-155.)

through the arthroscope to ensure that its integrity has been maintained and that there is no impingement of the graft in the intercondylar notch with knee range of motion. The knee is then copiously irrigated, and wounds are closed in a standard fashion.

Management and Outcome Summary

The patient's examination under anesthesia revealed a grade II Lachman test with a pseudoendpoint, a grade II anterior drawer test, and a grade II pivot-shift test, all of which were asymmetric compared with the opposite limb. The patient had no collateral ligament, PCL, or posterolateral corner laxity. Arthroscopic examination of the knee revealed a full-thickness peripheral tear of the posterior medial meniscus. In addition, the ACL was intact but vertically oriented to the 12 o'clock position on the femur (**Figure 12**). The tibial tunnel for the ACL graft was noted to be vertical and posterior.

The meniscal pathology was addressed with an inside-out suture technique. Attention was then directed to the ACL graft. The former tibial screw was removed, and there was no evidence of tunnel widening. The tibial guide was set at 55° and placed anterior to the former tibial tunnel. The new tibial tunnel was drilled, and some intra-articular overlap of the tibial tunnels was noted. Therefore, primary bone grafting of the former tibial tunnel was performed using autograft reamings from the new tibial tunnel.

Once the tibial tunnel was created, attention was turned to the femoral tunnel. An accessory transpatellar portal created during the index procedure was used to remove the femoral screw because trial placement of the femoral offset guide in the appropriate over-the-top position through the accessory inferomedial portal showed that the location of the screw interfered with proper femoral tunnel placement. No tunnel widening was noted during screw removal. The prior femoral tunnel was then filled with bone graft obtained from the allograft used for the reconstruction using a cut section of clear suction tubing placed retrograde through the tibial tunnel. By directing the tubing toward the prior femoral tunnel, extravasation of bone graft material into the joint was minimized. A new femoral tunnel was created endoscopically using the accessory inferomedial tunnel with the knee placed in hyperflexion. Adequate bone bridging was noted between the new and prior femoral tunnels. The graft was then placed retrograde into the knee joint using a push-in technique, and a 7- × 25-mm metal interference screw secured the graft to the femur. The knee was cycled multiple times with tension on the graft, and the tibial side of the graft was secured using a 9- × 20-mm metal interference screw. The Lachman, anterior drawer, and pivot-shift tests were normal after securing the graft.

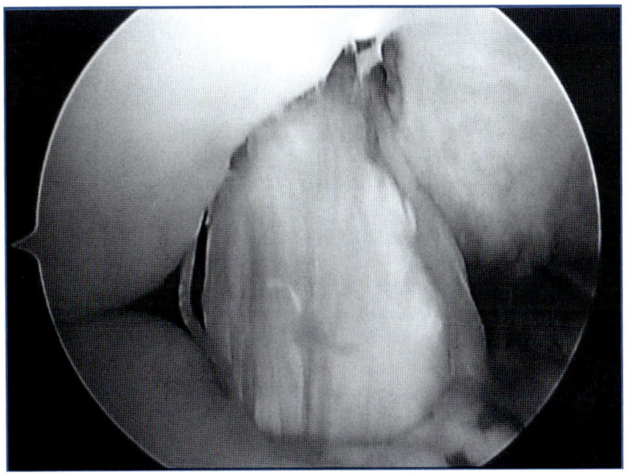

Figure 12 Arthroscopic image of a graft that is too vertically oriented on the femur and too posterior on the tibia results in a vertical graft that does not control rotation. Note that the graft tissue looks intact.

Radiographs taken postoperatively demonstrated a more anterior tibial tunnel and a femoral tunnel more laterally oriented at the 10:30 o'clock position (**Figure 13**). The patient had an uneventful postoperative course, and at 2 years KT-1000 arthrometric testing of both knees revealed a side-to-side left and right difference of 0 mm, 0 mm, and 0 mm with 15 lb, 20 lb, and maximum manual testing, respectively.

Strategies to Minimize Common Complications

Revision ACL reconstruction is a complex procedure that both the surgeon and the patient should view as a salvage procedure. Realistic expectations and a frank discussion about outcomes that are less predictable need to be communicated to the patient.

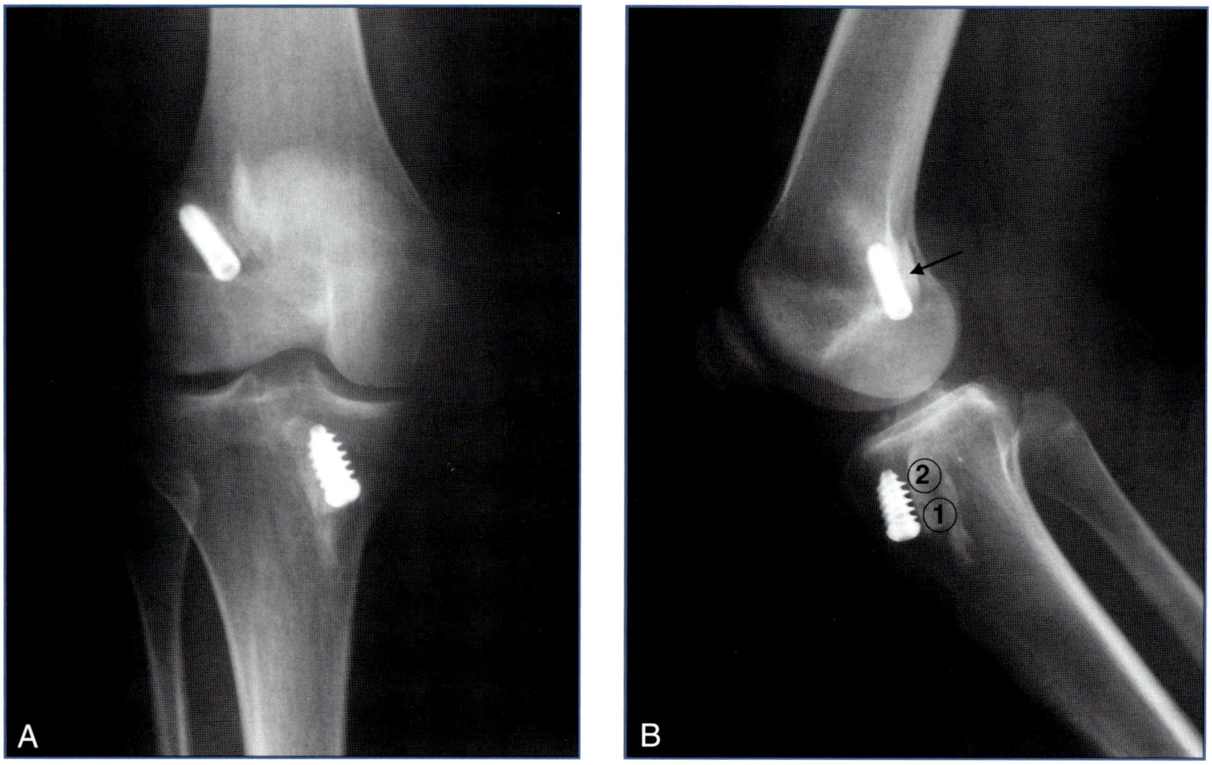

Figure 13 **A,** Postoperative AP radiograph shows a different orientation of the graft and femoral screw. **B,** Lateral radiograph shows the bone graft used to fill the vertically oriented femoral tunnel (arrow). On the tibia, the bone plug (2) directly posterior to the tibial interference screw is the revision graft that is "sandwiched" between the screw and the index reconstruction tibial bone plug, which was positioned too far posterior (1). (Part B is reproduced from Bach BR Jr, Fox JA, Mazzocca AD: Revision ACL reconstruction. *Orthopaedic Knowledge Online*. Rosemont, Illinois, American Academy of Orthopaedic Surgeons, 2002.)

Results of revision ACL reconstruction are affected by abnormal articular surfaces, meniscal deficiency, and the possibility of previously unrecognized associated patholaxities.

Preoperatively, the surgeon must determine whether the tunnels were created properly in the index procedure, whether they are anatomic or nonanatomic, and whether the tunnels are expanded. Expanded tunnels may require a staged procedure with bone grafting of the tunnels and a 4- to 6-month delay in ACL reconstruction. In addition, careful consideration about whether hardware placed at the time of the index procedure must be removed; a variety of screwdrivers and extraction instruments should be available at the time of the revision surgery.

Intraoperatively, the original intra-articular sites should be carefully exposed. If an allograft is being used, new tunnels are advised before the graft is prepared in the event that larger bone plugs may be required to compensate for slight tunnel overlap or tunnel expansion. After the femoral tunnel is created, the arthroscope should be advanced retrograde through the tibial tunnel up into the femoral socket to confirm that an intact femoral tunnel exists and that there has been no intratunnel blowout. If questions remain about the strength of graft fixation, supplemental fixation should be considered.

The postoperative course should be more conservative following revision ACL reconstruction than for the index procedure. Nevertheless, complete extension or hyperextension must be achieved postoperatively, as should patellar mobilization, to avoid scar formation and early quadriceps activity. Despite limited data on the timing for return to sport following revision ACL reconstruction, we believe that generally it should be delayed for at least 6 months postoperatively.

References

1. Williams RJ III, Warren RF, Carson EW, Wickiewicz TL: Revision anterior cruciate ligament reconstruction: The Hospital for Special Surgery experience. *Tech Orthop* 1998;12:375-383.
2. Steadman JR, Saterbak AM: Revision anterior cruciate ligament reconstruction: Technique and tips. The Vail experience. *Tech Orthop* 1998;13:384-390.
3. Clancy WG Jr, Peitropaoli MP: Revision anterior cruciate ligament reconstruction using the "anatomic-endoscopic" method. *Tech Orthop* 1998;13:391-410.
4. Bach BR Jr., Mazzocca A, Fox JA: Revision anterior cruciate ligament surgery, in Grana WA (ed): *Orthopaedic Knowledge Online*. Rosemont, IL, American Academy of Orthopaedic Surgeons, 2003. Available at www.aaos.org/oko.
5. Noyes FR, Barber-Westin SD: Revision anterior cruciate ligament reconstruction: Report of 11-year experience and results in 114 consecutive patients. *Instr Course Lect* 2001;50:451-461.
6. Bach BR Jr, Jones GT, Sweet FA, Hager CA: Arthroscopically-assisted anterior cruciate ligament reconstruction using patellar tendon substitution: Two- to four-year follow-up results. *Am J Sports Med* 1994;22:758-767.
7. Bach BR Jr, Levy ME, Bojchuk J, Tradonsky S, Bush-Joseph CA, Khan NH:. Single-incision endoscopic anterior cruciate ligament reconstruction using patellar tendon autograft: Minimum two-year follow-up evaluation. *Am J Sports Med* 1998;26:30-40.
8. Bach BR Jr, Tradonsky S, Bojchuk J, Levy ME, Bush-Joseph CA, Khan NH: Arthroscopically assisted anterior cruciate ligament reconstruction using patellar tendon autograft: Five- to nine-year follow-up evaluation. *Am J Sports Med* 1998;26:20-29.
9. Bach BR Jr: Revision ACL reconstruction: Indications and technique, in Miller M, Cole B (eds): *Textbook of Arthroscopy*. Philadelphia, PA, Saunders-Elsevier, 2004, pp 675-686.
10. Bach BR Jr: Revision anterior cruciate ligament surgery. *Arthroscopy* 2003;19(suppl 1): 14-19.
11. Fideler BM, Vangsness CT Jr, Lu B, et al: Gamma irradiation: Effects on biomechanical properties of human bone-patellar tendon-bone allografts. *Am J Sports Med* 1995;23:643-646.
12. Curran AR, Adams DJ, Gill JL, Steiner ME, Scheller AD: The biomechanical effects of low-dose irradiation on bone-patellar tendon-bone allografts. *Am J Sports Med* 2004;32:1131-1135.
13. Noyes FR, Barber-Westin SD: Revision anterior cruciate surgery with use of bone-patellar tendon-bone autogenous grafts. *J Bone Joint Surg Am* 2001;83:1131-1143.
14. Bach BR Jr: Observations on interference screw morphologies. *Arthroscopy* 2000;16:E10. Available at www.arthroscopy-journal.org.
15. O'Donnell JB, Scerpella TA: Endoscopic anterior cruciate ligament reconstruction: Modified technique and radiographic review. *Arthroscopy* 1995;11:577-584.

INDEX

Page numbers with *f* indicate figure

A

Adhesive band excision, 41
Anterior cortical disruption, 15
Anterior cruciate ligament (ACL)
  bone-patellar-bone grafts, 14*f*
  failed reconstruction, 49-59
  incompetence, 65
  preoperative evaluation, 55-56
  revision, 22*f*
    extensor compromise, 21-28
    failed, 49-59
    graft fixation, 9-19
    graft harvest, 1-7
    patellar fracture, 21-28
    septic arthritis, 29-34
    technical aspects, 61-73
    two-incision revision technique, 13*f*
  rupture, 10*f*
  tears
    acute, 50*f*
    chronic, 51*f*
    midsubstance, 2*f*
Anti-inflammatory medication (NSAIDs), 36
Arthrofibrosis
  after ACL reconstruction, 35-48
  arthroscopic débridement, 40-41
  biologic graft failure and, 54
  classification, 37-38
  definition, 36-37
  management of, 40-44
  mechanism of injury, 39-40
  prevention of, 44
  recognition of, 36-39
  risk factors, 39-40
  surgical outcomes, 46
  timing of surgery, 39, 44-45
Arthroscopic débridement
  algorithm, 43*f*
  arthrofibrosis, 40-41
  patient positioning, 41*f*

B

Beath pin placement, 9
Bone bruises, 10*f*
Bone grafts
  extravasation, 72
  harvest site, 25
  matchstick technique, 69, 70*f*
  overlapping tunnels and, 62, 63*f*
  piggyback technique, 3*f*
Bone-patellar tendon-bone (BTB) grafts, 14*f*
  graft-construct mismatch, 15-16
  graft fixation problems, 9-19
  irrigation and débridement, 30*f*
  revision, 57*f*
  septic arthritis after, 29-34

Bone plugs
double, 56-57
femoral placement, 62*f*
fracture of, 1, 3*f*
geometry, 25
graft preparation, 68-71
inadequate, 6
interface with screws, 15
removal technique, 6, 25
salvage options, 15
tibial, 62*f*
undersized, 3
Bone-to-bone healing, 54
Bone-to-tendon healing, 54
Bracing, 22, 25, 26, 42

C

C-reactive protein, 31, 32
Chondrolysis, 31, 33*f*
Chopat strap, 26
Cobb elevators, 68
Complex regional pain syndrome (CRPS), 39, 40
Contamination of grafts, 5-6
Continuous passive motion devices, 32, 42
Cross-pin fixation, 3
Cyclops lesions, 36, 37*f*, 38, 39, 42*f*

D

Débridement instruments, 65
Devascularization, 26

E

Effusion, 55
Electrocautery, 65
EndoButton, 12, 17*f*, 17-18, 30, 32
Extensor mechanism
arthrofibrosis and, 36
compromise, 21-28
graft selection, 45
macrotraumatic complications, 24
risks to, 2
Extracapsular fibrosis, 37

F

Femoral condyles
bone bruise, 10*f*
flattening, 33*f*
impingement, 52, 53*f*
scar adherence, 37*f*
Femoral guides
J-shaped passer, 12, 13*f*
rear-entry, 14*f*, 68
Femoral sockets
drilling, 12*f*
EndoButton insertion, 17*f*
posterior wall blowout, 9-19, 10*f*, 67
rear-entry guide, 18*f*
Femoral tunnels, 66-68
expansion, 63*f*
graft preparation, 69
grafting, 72
inferomedial portal, 67*f*
nonoverlapping, nonanatomic, 63*f*
placement, 11-13, 52, 52*f*, 53*f*, 67*f*
posterior cortex violation, 68*f*
vertically oriented, 71
Fibrous hyperplasia, 38
Flexion contractures, 36, 38
Fluoroscopy, 66
Free bone block technique, 16*f*
"Funnel" concept, 64, 64*f*

G

Graft-construct mismatch, 15-16, 16*f*
Grafts
arthrofibrosis and, 39
biologic failure, 54
contamination, 5-6
fixation, 9-19
fixation failure, 54
harvest complications, 1-7
impingement, 38, 53-54
improper orientation, 71*f*
ligament deficiencies, 54-55
premature amputation, 2
selection, 65
tension, 39, 53
traumatic failure, 54

Guide pins
- drilling, 13*f*
- femoral insertion, 11, 68
- removal, 67
- tibial, 53*f*, 65, 66

H
Hamstrings tendons
- fixation complications, 17-18
- harvest, 2, 4*f*, 4-5, 6
- stripping, 5

Hardware removal, 66
Hemostasis, 41

I
Immobilization, 38, 40. *see also* Rehabilitation
Infections, 39, 40, 54. *see also* Septic arthritis
Inferomedial portal, 67*f*
Inflammation
- arthrofibrosis and, 39, 44
- development of, 42-43
- posttraumatic, 45

Infrapatellar contracture syndrome, 37, 38*f*
Inside-out approaches, 63*f*
Intercondylar notch, 41, 50*f*
Interference screws
- ACL reconstruction with, 51*f*
- bioabsorbable, 15, 18
- breakage, 15
- compromised fixation, 11
- fixation using, 12, 15
- placement, 12, 14*f*
- removal, 67*f*
- soft-tissue fixation, 3
- stacked, 70*f*
- tibial, 32

J
Joint line tenderness, 55
Joint space narrowing, 33*f*

K
Kirschner wires (K-wires), 24
Knee
- hyperextension, 36
- medial anatomy, 4*f*
- stiffness issues, 43-44
- varus alignment, 54

Kocher clamps, 66, 66*f*
Krackow sutures, 3, 15

L
Lachman test, 53, 69
Lag screws, transverse, 24
Lateral collateral ligaments (LCL), 12
Ligaments. see also specific Ligaments
- deficiencies, 54-55
- testing, 55

M
Marshall-MacIntosh procedure, 26
Matchstick technique, 69, 70*f*
McLaughlin-type wire, 26
Medial collateral ligament (MCL)
- repair, 40
- risk to, 5
- superficial, 4

Meniscus
- lateral, 22
- medial, 50, 54, 57*f*
- tears, 22, 39, 50*f*, 56
- transplant, 50, 54, 56-57

N
Neurapraxia, 39
Notchplasty, 39, 65

O
Oscillating saw, 6
Osgood-Schlatter disease, 16
Ossification, accessory, 16
Osteonecrosis, zone of, 33*f*
Osteopenia, secondary, 24
Osteophytes, 33*f*, 39
Osteotomes, 25
Outside-in approaches, 63*f*

P

Patella baja, 16, 37-38
Patella infera, 37-38
Patella
  fractures, 21-28
    fixation, 24*f*
    longitudinal, 24, 24*f*
    management, 24-25
    postoperative, 23*f*
    prevention, 25
    reduction, 23*f*
    rehabilitation, 24-25
  mobility, 42
  size of, 2
Patellar tendinitis, 26-27
Patellar tendons, 70*f*
  fixation, 16*f*
  graft selection, 45
  harvest, 1-2, 3-4, 6, 65
  inadequate length, 16
  insertion, 4*f*
  narrow, 3
  rupture, 25-26
Patellofemoral joint, 36
Pivot-shift test, 69
Posterior cruciate ligament (PCL), 52, 67
Posterior wall, examination, 12*f*
Posterior wall blowout, 9-19, 11-12, 67
Postoperative motion recovery, 46*f*
Preoperative evaluation, 65
Pyarthrosis, 31

Q

Quadriceps inhibition, 38

R

Range of motion
  arthrofibrosis and, 39, 40
  exercises, 42
Reamers
  advancement, 13f, 67
  cannulated, 68
  for EndoButton insertion, 17
Rear-entry guide, 18*f*
Rehabilitation
  after patellar fracture fixation, 24-25
  after septic arthritis, 32
  arthrofibrosis and, 39, 40, 41-43
  brace protection and, 25
  patellar tendinitis and, 26
  postoperative, 45-46
  traumatic graft failure and, 54

S

Scar tissue
  arthrofibrosis and, 36
  débridement, 41
  excision, 41
  suprapatellar pouch, 37*f*, 42*f*
Screw-and-washer constructs, 15
Semitendinosus tendons
  accessory bands, 5
  exposure, 5
  harvest, 4
  premature amputation, 6
  premature cut, 2, 2*f*
Septic arthritis
  ACL reconstruction and, 29-34
  graft removal, 32
  graft retention and, 31-32
  irrigation and débridement, 30*f*
  management, 31-32
  signs and symptoms, 30
  Sinding-Larsen-Johansson disease, 16
Single-incision technique, 70*f*
Soft tissue
  fixation, 3, 3*f*
  inflammation, 39
Staphylococcus aureus, 30, 31
Staphylococcus epidermis, 31
Staple fixation, 15
Stress shielding, 54
Suprapatellar pouch, 37, 42*f*
Suture passers, J-shaped, 13*f*

T

Tendon strippers, 2, 5*f*
Terminal extension, blocks to, 38-39

Tibia
- bone plug, 62*f*
- osteophyte, 39*f*
- proximal, 4*f*

Tibial aimer, 66*f*
Tibial guide pins, 65, 66
Tibial tunnels, 65-66
- expansion, 63*f*
- graft preparation, 69
- grafting of, 72
- malposition, 14-15
- placement, 10, 52, 64
- reaming, 15

Tunnels. *see also* Femoral tunnels; Tibial tunnels
- compromise of, 10
- expansion, 65
- graft-construct mismatch, 15-16

Two-incision technique
- ACL reconstruction, 51*f*, 64-65
- conversion to, 12
- femoral tunnel, 68*f*
- incisions, 67, 68*f*
- rear-entry instruments, 13*f*

V
Vascularity, inadequate, 54

W
Weight bearing in extension, 46
Wound healing, 55

Z
Z-knee retractors, 67-68